# A
# CRUCIFIX

REV. DR. MARLENE LOUISE WALTERS

WESTBOW
PRESS®
A DIVISION OF THOMAS NELSON
& ZONDERVAN

WestBow Press books may be ordered through booksellers or by contacting:

WestBow Press
A Division of Thomas Nelson & Zondervan
1663 Liberty Drive
Bloomington, IN 47403
www.westbowpress.com
844-714-3454

Scripture taken from the New King James Version®. Copyright © 1982 by Thomas Nelson. Used by permission. All rights reserved.

ISBN: 978-1-6642-4739-0 (sc)
ISBN: 978-1-6642-4740-6 (hc)
ISBN: 978-1-6642-4741-3 (e)

Library of Congress Control Number: 2021921014

Print information available on the last page.

WestBow Press rev. date: 11/11/2021

# Contents

# Contents

*A Crucifix* is a true story of a unique heirloom given to the author of this book and the adventure it presented to unveil the reason this unexpected and curious visitor gave it to her.

The odyssey expands through years of anecdotes from the life and experiences of the writer as she attempts to disclose the mystery of this unexpected keepsake.

Reverend Doctor Marlene Louise Walters encountered several experiences that led to attending and graduating from Palmer Theological Seminary (PTS) with a Master of Divinity degree. Later, she received her doctorate at PTS, with her dissertation title, "Sanctity or Quality of Life." Dr. Walters is an ordained United Methodist minister and founder and facilitator of numerous support groups. She served as a hospital chaplain and a minister at Grace United Methodist Church; Mt. Lebanon United Methodist Church in Wilmington, Delaware; and a Chapel community in Florida.

Teaching medical ethics to interns at the Medical Center of Wilmington, Delaware, and students at Eastern College in St. Davids, Pennsylvania; Washington College in Chestertown, Maryland; and the Nursing School of Wilmington gave her a unique ability to question and debate issues such as abortion, euthanasia, suicide, living wills, hospice, and doctor- or physician-assisted suicide.

These dilemmas are also present in this book, *A Crucifix*.

Marlene and Tom just celebrated their sixty-eighth wedding anniversary, with their three children, six grandchildren, and one great-grandson. Tom and Marlene are living in a retirement community at St. Simons Island, Georgia.

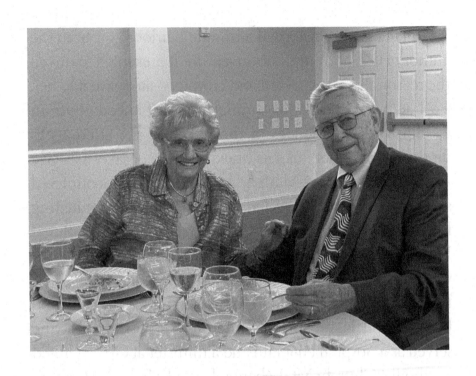

======================================

This book, *A Crucifix*, is dedicated to my dearest friend, ardent supporter, caring husband, loving father of our children, endearing grandfather and great-grandfather, patriot of our beloved country, outstanding architect and planner, and spiritual mate:

Colonel Thomas J. Walters A.I.A (American Institute Architects)

======================================

# Chapter 1
## "Dr. J."

As our lives draw to a close, the disposition and equal distribution of our belongings becomes an issue for our family.

What should I to do with the crucifix that Dr. J gave to me?

Tom and I had just finished breakfast and were sitting on our back screened-in porch.

Then the phone rang.

Rather than write his real name, I'll give him an assumed name: "Dr. J."

"Dr. J." asked if I would be home, as he wanted to bring me something.

I said, "Yes." It would be nice to see him, although I hardly recalled his name, but I did remember his wife. I'll use a pseudonym, "Iris." However, "Iris" and I had many differing beliefs about the abortion, living will, and doctor-assisted-suicide issues. I am pro-life, and Iris is pro-choice on most medical ethical questions.

When Dr. J. arrived at our home, I honestly didn't remember his thin, bent-over osteoporotic appearance, but then I hadn't seen him in years, except I knew he was a revered Delaware pediatrician.

My husband, Tom, and I invited him in, but he wanted to sit on our screened-in porch. He talked for a few minutes, but neither Tom nor I can remember our conversation; it was so short.

He reached into his pocket with his slender hands,

pulled out a blue jewelry box, and opened it to small fragile black box inside. It was then he lifted this delicate crucifix, attached to an antique necklace, and tenderly handed it to me.

Dr. J. gently said, "My family gave this to me, and I give it to you."

I was speechless. I didn't know what to say, except, "Thank you."

Of course, I smiled as I carefully took the crucifix from his hand to mine. I was going to put it on, but Dr. J. stood up and once again gave his hand to me, as he moved to the screened-in porch door.

I wanted to run after him and ask him, "Why me?" but Dr. J. left, as he obviously didn't want to engage in any further conversation. He stated that he wanted to give me his "family crucifix." On the back of the crucifix was etched "BM 1827," and on the left were these words, etched in French, "Gage D'amitie." Searching on Google, I found the meaning of "Gage D'amitie: "token of friendship."

The crucifix was approximately two inches by an inch and half in size and solid gold with a black enamel inset.

Inside the box that held the crucifix and chain on a green folded piece of paper were these words:

"Cross given to, Countess Rehbender [Unsure of spelling: could be Rchbender] Berlin."

Then was the name of "Dr. J." in 1942 and "Given to Marlene Walters by Dr. J. 1994."

I searched through Ancestory.com for the name of Countess Rehbender, but neither that name nor Rchbender was anywhere to be found.

Then, a few months after Dr. J. so kindly brought his precious gift to me, I found his name in the *Wilmington News Journal's* obituary page.

I couldn't believe it. Dr. J. had died, and I didn't know him. He called my house, came to my home, and presented me his family crucifix.

He had to know me.

Why would Dr. J. give me his precious heirloom, a crucifix? Why, indeed?

========================================

As Tom and I vocally try to determine where Dr. J. and I crossed paths, I begin my mental journey.

When we first moved to Delaware from Ft. Leonard Wood, Missouri, where my husband served in the US Army, we needed a pediatrician for our daughters.

Dr. J.'s practice was so well known and busy that when I called his office to sign up, they were at their limit in accepting new patients.

So, Dr. J. didn't know our family in his private practice. If not there, where?

What a mystery for us to unfold. Even though I don't remember seeing him, he must've met or known me from somewhere. Why else would he have given me such a lovely keepsake as his crucifix?

I doubt he knew me in my "before ministry" life, as I always called it. I was a mother of three, wife, and volunteer for the Easter Seal Society, American Red Cross, John G. Leach School, and Mancus Foundation. My main emphasis in all those organizations was working with disabled children. However, during those years, I was in my early thirties, and Dr. J. gave me his crucifix when I

**was sixty-one years old. I doubt he knew me in my-before ministry years.**

**Perhaps I met him in 1969 when I was thirty-six years old and in Dover, Delaware, unwillingly witnessing the first abortion bill in the State of Delaware.**

==========================================

Why was I in the Dover, Delaware, Legislative Hall in 1969?

I was teaching swimming for special-ed children from the John G. Leach School in the state of Delaware.

The kids, many of whom couldn't move their arms and legs, were delighted to enter the warm waters of the heated swimming pool. It was in that atmosphere of tepid temperatures that the disabled person feels his or her muscles relax and is frequently actually able to move.

"Look at me, Mrs. Walters. I can move!" was the often-heard exclamation by my students.

Why did I like teaching the disabled kids? Hearing those appreciative responses, knowing they really did understand gratitude and thanksgiving, whereas most of us who have been gifted with normal physical bodies take our movable limbs for granted.

One day, I was approached by a Junior League friend, whose husband was a Delaware politician. She asked me, "Would you bring some of the disabled children down to the capital of Delaware? We really need you all to help us at an upcoming important hearing. Will you come and bring a couple of the handicapped kids?"

We had been working hard on getting handicapped

ramps put in the many state-owned buildings, so I thought we might finally be getting our hearing for handicap-accessible ramps.

"Yes, of course," I replied.

"Don't forget to get permission slips from the parents," she advised.

With two permission slips in hand, two of my handicapped children and I traveled to Dover, about an hour's drive from Wilmington, Delaware. When I emptied the van and entered the colonial capital building, the kids were joyfully singing, "We're going to get our ramps. Yippee."

Then it was time for my politician friend to start the hearing, and he nodded for me to wheel my kids around the Legislative Hall. "Ladies and Gentlemen of Delaware, we must pass this Senate Bill Number 200 that will allow women to abort their fetus if they're known to have a handicap."

*What? Shock!*

"Does anyone object?" intoned an unfamiliar voice from the chamber floor.

No one answered, and my throat was caught in glue. How could I speak? I had never spoken in public before. What would I say to these people who obviously never swam with, sat with, talked with, or cared for a handicapped-disabled person?

So, I gathered the special needs kids and went directly to the van, without uttering a word. On the way home, one of the kids spoke enthusiastically, "Mrs. Walters, are we gonna get our ramps now? Did I do good?"

No, the Senate bill wasn't for ramps but shockingly allowing an abortion of a handicapped infant.

I leaned my chin on my left shoulder so they wouldn't see tears flowing from my eyes as I drove back to the John G. Leach School. How could I know the trip to the capital was for aborting handicapped kids and not for putting in ramps?

And then, I said something that led me on a fifty-year journey with myself, God, and whoever else would listen, including my husband and three children.

"Oh, God, forgive me that I said nothing. What can I do? Please lead me."

Amazingly the next day, there were two advertisements in the *Wilmington News Journal*: "Lancaster Theological Seminary is waiting for you" and "Come visit Eastern Baptist Theological Seminary" (EBTS). These ads seemed to jump out of the newspaper in front of my eyes. I knew I had to do something but what? I got in my Mustang the next day and drove to Lancaster, Pennsylvania. The following day, I visited EBTS, now known as Palmer Theological Seminary, in the suburbs of Philadelphia.

Both seminaries wanted me to enroll in their Master of Divinity program. However, I decided on EBTS because it was only a forty-five-minute ride, whereas LTS was over an hour away.

At EBTS, I met Dr. Norman Maring, the Christian history professor, who encouraged me to sign up for a class as the first woman of my age entering the master of divinity degree program. Here I was a thirty-six-year-old woman, wife of sixteen years with my husband, Tom, and mother of three daughters, Debbie, Becky, and Carrie, one teenager, one preteenager, and one in elementary school, all needing me.

Yikes.

*What am I doing going to seminary? How will I be able to balance my precious children, my good husband, and my already full life with the new life that will be filled with reading many books, tests, exams, and all that goes with the desire to get a ninety-six-hour master of divinity degree?*

Not only that but my husband, Tom, and I didn't have extra money for my schooling, as we were saving for our children's education. When I approached him, asking if I could go to seminary, the answer was absolutely "No! We're saving up money only for our daughters' educations!" Then he asked the poignant question, "How will your going to seminary change the abortion issue?"

And he was right. What was I doing and why? I wasn't sure what I was doing, as all of my female friends were proabortion. They felt a woman had a right to her own body and should be the only one making the decision about whether she could have an abortion or not—no input from the father or anyone else.

"What about taking the life of a person?" I would ask.

"The fetus is not a person yet," would be the usual response.

Then, what is "it"? As I poured over any scientific books I could find in the library, I wondered, "When is a person a person?"

I made appointments with several Protestant ministers, priests, and a rabbi. All but the priests felt it was up to the woman to decide, at least up to the time of viability, about the twenty-fourth week of pregnancy.

The priests thought a baby was a human at the time of conception.

Most of them believed a pregnant woman could abort her baby if it resulted from incest or rape.

==========================================

**Now I'm wondering, did I meet Dr. J. at that abortion hearing? As I reflect on that original 1969 abortion bill and how that day changed my life forever, I don't think that my crucifix-giving Dr. J. was in Dover, Delaware.**

**However, I do believe he had an interest in the abortion debate because his wife was a politician, and she favored abortion on demand.**

==========================================

# Chapter 2
## Jesus: The Feminist

I really needed to find out more about my Lord and Savior, Jesus. After all, I wouldn't want to be ordained if it was true that Jesus didn't want women to preach His word.

How did Jesus treat women? What does the Holy Bible say? As I began my research, I wondered if Jesus said or did anything that would indicate that he advocated treating women as intrinsically inferior to men. What I found was that Jesus said and did things that indicated He thought of women as equals to men and that, in the process, He willingly violated pertinent social mores.

Let me explain.

There were very important factors and laws in existence during Jesus's time that were quite significant.

How were women treated? What was the status of women in Palestine? During the time of Jesus, women were treated as inferiors. According to most rabbinic customs of Jesus's time, women were not allowed to study the scriptures, the Torah.

In the virtually religious area of prayer, women, along with children and slaves, were not allowed to recite the Schema or prayers at any meals. In fact, the Talmud states, "Let a curse come upon the man whose wife or children says grace for him." In the great worship temple at Jerusalem, women were limited to the outer portion, the women's court, which was five steps below the court for children. Besides the ostracizing women suffered in the areas of prayer and worship, there were other restrictions in the private and public forums of that society. It was thought disreputable to speak to women in public. The Proverbs of the Fathers contained the injunction "Speak not with a woman in public." It was written in public documents, "who speaks much with a woman draws down misfortune on himself, neglects the word of the law and finally earns hell."

It sure wasn't easy being born a woman in those days. In addition, save the rarest instance, women were not allowed to bear witness in a court of law.

Some thinkers in that era, Philio, a contemporary of Jesus, for example, wrote that, "women ought not leave their households, girls ought not cross the threshold that separated the male and female apartments of the household." In general, the attitude toward women was epitomized in the institution and customs surrounding marriage.

For the most part, the function of women was thought rather exclusively in terms of childbearing and rearing.

Women were almost always under the tutelage of a man, either the father or husband or, if a widow, the dead husband's brother. Polygamy, in the sense of having several wives but not in the sense of having several husbands, was legal at the time Jesus walked the earth. Divorce of a wife was very easily obtained by the husband. He merely had to give her a writ of divorce. Women in Palestine, in contrast, were not allowed to divorce their husbands.

Rabbinic sayings—and remember Jesus was a Jew and a rabbi—provide an insight into their attitudes toward women. One of these sayings was "It is well for those whose children who are male, but ill for those whose children are female."

10

Even the most virtuous of women have four qualities. They are greedy at their food, eager to gossip, lazy, and jealous."

The condition of women in Palestine was indeed bleak.

With this in mind, I began to look at the good book, the Holy Bible, especially when our Lord walked the earth.

What are the gospels?

The first four books of the New Testament, Matthew, Mark, Luke, and John are eyewitness reports of the events in the life of Jesus of Nazareth. They are four different faith statements reflecting four primitive Christian communities who believed that Jesus was the Messiah and Savior of the world.

They were composed from a variety of sources, written and oral, over a period of time. Consequently, they are many layered.

What's important to remember is the fact that no negative attitudes by Jesus toward women are portrayed in the gospels. When you set them side by side with the disrespectful treatment of women of those times, it's amazing to see how Jesus treated women.

When I began my journey, the word *feminist* was just beginning to emerge. Being a feminist really means a person who is in favor and promotes the equality of women with men.

One of the first things I noticed in the gospels about Jesus's attitude toward women is that He taught them the meaning of scripture and religious truths in general.

When you remember that in Judaism, it was considered improper and even "obscene" to teach women the scriptures, this action of Jesus was an extraordinary and deliberate decision to break with a custom invidious to women.

A number of women, married and unmarried, were regular followers of Jesus.

"Jesus made his way through towns and villages preaching and proclaiming the good news of the Kingdom of God. With Him went the twelve as well as certain women who provided for them out of their own resources" (Luke 8:1–3).

Jesus's first appearance after His resurrection to any of His followers was to two women: Mary Magdalene and the other Mary from whom Jesus cast out seven demons.

These women were commissioned by Jesus to bear witness of His resurrection to the eleven disciples, which is recorded in three of the gospels: John 20:11; Matthew 28:5 and Mark 16:9.

And, in typical Palestinian style, the eleven disciples refused to believe the women. Remember, according to Judaic law, women were not allowed to bear legal witness. As one learned in the law, Jesus obviously was aware of this stricture.

Jesus first appearing to and commissioning women to be a witness to the most important event of His career, His resurrection, couldn't have been anything but deliberate.

Other intimate connections concerning women and resurrections are also written in the gospels.

The first account is that of the raising of a woman, Jairus's daughter, recorded in three gospels: Matthew 9:18, Mark 5:33, and Luke 8:41.

The second resurrection Jesus performed was that of the only son of the widow of Nain. "And when the Lord saw her, He had compassion on her and said, 'Be well,' and He touched the casket and said, 'arise,' and Jesus delivered him to his mother, and all were amazed" (Luke 7:11).

The third resurrection Jesus performed was of Lazarus, at the request of Lazarus's sisters, Mary and Martha, from the gospel (John 11:1–29).

From the first, it was Martha and Mary who had sent for Jesus, but when He finally came, Lazarus was dead four days. Martha met Jesus and pleaded for Lazarus's resurrection. "Lord, if you had been here, my brother would not have died and even now I know that whatever you ask from God, God will give you" (John 11:21). And then He raised Lazarus from the dead, and immediately following, Jesus declared himself to be the resurrection.

To Martha, Jesus said, "I am the resurrection and the life. He who believes in Me, though he may die, he shall live. And, whoever lives and believes in Me, shall never die. Do you believe this?"

And Martha said to Jesus, "Yes, Lord, I believe that You are the Christ, the Son of God, who is to come into the world" (John 11:24, 25).

Jesus once again revealed the central event, the central message in the gospels—the resurrection—to a woman.

In other places in the gospel where women were treated by others not as persons but as sexual objects, it was expected Jesus would do the same.

Their expectations were disappointed.

One such occasion occurred when Jesus was invited to dinner at the house of a skeptical Pharisee. There was a woman known to be of ill repute who washed Jesus's feet with her tears and anointed them.

The Pharisee saw her only as an evil creature. But Jesus deliberately rejected this approach of the woman as a sinner. Jesus rebuked the Pharisee and spoke of her love and her being forgiven, and then Jesus addressed her. Remember, it was not proper to speak to a woman in public, especially an improper woman.

Jesus spoke to her as a human being. He said to the woman, "Your faith has saved you. Go in Peace" (Luke 7:50).

A similar situation occurred when the Scribes and Pharisees used a woman reduced entirely as a sex object to set a legal trap for Jesus. The woman was caught in adultery, and the Pharisees asked Jesus about the Law of Moses that commanded them that the woman should be stoned.

It is difficult to imagine a more callous use of a human person than the "adulterous" woman being placed by the enemies of Jesus.

First, she was surprised in the intimate act of sexual intercourse and then dragged before the Scribes and Pharisees and an even larger crowd that Jesus was instructing, making her stand in full view of everybody. The Scribes and Pharisees told Jesus that she had been caught in the very act of committing adultery.

They reminded Jesus that Moses had commanded that such a woman be stoned to death. The Pharisees asked Jesus, "What do you have to say?" (John 9:5).

The trap was partly that if Jesus said, "Yes," to the stoning, He would be violating the Roman law, which

14

restricted capital punishment, and if Jesus said, "No," He would appear to contravene Mosaic Law.

Jesus eluded their snares by refusing to become entangled in legalisms and abstractions.

Rather, He dealt with both the accusers and the accused directly as spiritual ethical human persons. Jesus spoke directly to the accusers in the context of their own personal ethical conduct.

Jesus said, "he who is without sin among you, let him throw a stone at her first" (John 8:7).

To the accused woman, He likewise spoke directly with compassion but without approving her conduct: "Woman where are those accusers of yours? Has no one condemned you?"

She said, "No, not one, Lord."

And Jesus said, "Neither do I condemn you. Go and do not sin again" (John 8:10, 11).

Now, remember the law concerning divorce at the time Jesus walked in Jerusalem. A man could write a writ of divorce for any reason, and the wife had to leave the home.

What does Jesus say about divorce? The Pharisees tempted Jesus, saying, "Is it lawful for a man to divorce his wife for just any reason?" (Matthew 19:3).

And Jesus answered, "Have you not read that He who made them in the beginning, made them male and female, and said, 'for this reason a man shall leave his father and mother and be joined to his wife, and the two shall become one flesh?'" (Matthew 19:4, 5).

And the Pharisees asked, "Why then did Moses

command to give a certificate of divorce and to put her away?"

Jesus said to them, "Moses, because of the hardness of your hearts, permitted you to divorce your wives, but from the beginning it was not so. And, I say to you, whoever divorces his wife, except for sexual immorality, and marries another, commits adultery; and whoever marries her who is divorced commits adultery" (Matthew 19:8, 9).

Again, when I recalled the Palestinian restriction on women studying the scriptures or studying with the rabbis, it is difficult to imagine how Jesus could have possibly been clearer, that women were called to the spiritual life just as men were.

In many ways, Jesus strove to communicate the notion of equality.

I was finding the gospel lessons of Jesus were, as I thought and was taught from my early Sunday school years, that Jesus accepts all people regardless of their gender, their color, or their handicap. All are unconditionally loved.

Now, after my research, I was feeling comfortable going to seminary, learning how to be a minister, and trying to find God in everyone I met.

I believe it's okay to be a woman and answer God's call.

====================================

**Dr. J. must have believed women could be ordained clergy too.**

**Why would he have given me his treasured crucifix if he didn't believe women could be preaching the word, serving Communion, and leading the church as a minister?**

I'm fortunate that I chose United Methodism as my denomination because our founder, John Wesley, was the first within his movement to authorize a woman to preach. In 1761, he granted a license to preach to Sarah Crosby. Wesley's appreciation for the importance of women in the church has been credited to his mother, Susanna Wesley, who instilled in John and his brother Charles a deep appreciation for the intellectual and spiritual qualities of women.

Choosing the Master of Divinity degree over the Master of Arts in Religion degree was a difficult one for me. I wanted to participate in God's world by becoming ordained. I really didn't understand why it was okay, as a woman, to be a Sunday school superintendent and teacher but not okay to be preaching God's word or delivering His Holy Communion elements.

More than frequently, people would ask me, "Haven't you read St. Paul's admonition against women, 'I do not permit a woman to teach or have authority over a man but to be in silence. Let a woman learn in silence with all submission.'"

Yes, Paul did say that in 1 Timothy 2:12. But you must remember, in Paul's era, women weren't even allowed inside the church. In those days, women were only allowed to sit on the circle outside the synagogue, behind the children.

When Paul said, "Let a woman learn in silence," he was giving women a chance to *learn* in silence, something she was not allowed to do before. At least Paul was allowing women to *enter and learn in silence*, which was a commemorative statement for a man of those times.

Many people were against women advancing in their chosen careers too. Yet it was the women who became bank managers and school superintendents and held

17

other lofty positions that allowed me to finally get my elder orders.

Let me explain.

To become a deacon, you had to be approved and recommended from your home church and then complete forty hours of the Master of Divinity degree at a seminary. That's about half the seminary credits needed to complete a Master of Divinity degree.

After becoming a deacon, which I received in 1976, the next step was elder, with the promise of always some kind of church employment as a full clergy in the United Methodist Church.

In the United Methodist *Book of Discipline*, all those hopeful clergymen waiting to become elders in their conferences must say, "I will," to several questions.

One of the questions was "Will you agree to be transferred whenever requested?"

If you wanted to become ordained, your answer had to be "yes." However, in my household, my dearly beloved husband, who had tolerated but not supported financially or emotionally my desire to become a minister by going to seminary, put his foot down at that question.

Tom's response? "I will not be transferred. If you want to be transferred, you'll have to go without me. I'm staying right here at 2424 Grubb Road and nowhere else!"

End of story.

He had condoned everything else but not being transferred. After all, our three daughters attended school close by with all their friends, and his office building was only a few miles away, as were many of his clients.

"I won't move," he declared.

Unless I wanted a divorce, when I was invited to speak to the Board of Ministry of the United Methodist hierarchy, I had to say, "No, I won't be transferred."

So, they dismissed me, not offering my elder orders

that would give me responsibilities to preach, teach, and preside at the celebration of the sacraments, administer the church through pastoral guidance, and lead congregations to service ministry.

I was devastated because I had worked so hard to get my deacon orders and was about to graduate magna cum laude with my Master of Divinity degree from Palmer Theological Seminary (EBTS).

I was fortunate to still have my position as a chaplain at the Wilmington Medical Center, but the Peninsula Delaware Conference didn't recognize me as a "clergyman." I mean *clergyperson*.

I had to wait another year to reapply, but I knew Tom wasn't going to change his position on being transferred, and I appreciated and agreed to his proclamation.

The next year, I resubmitted my desire to receive my elder orders, as I'd graduated and was still volunteering as a hospital chaplain, but now the Medical Center was paying for my tuition into the Doctor of Ministry degree at my seminary.

I was called into the grim room of all older men, and once again, I told them I wouldn't answer "yes" to the "Will you be transferred?" question.

Amazingly, they agreed that I wouldn't have to be transferred. In fact, they'd reconsidered that question.

Why? Because the male candidates for elder orders had wives whose careers elevated them to high positions in their companies, banks, and schools, and they didn't want to be transferred either.

Women did it again.

Thank heavens clergymen's wives were advancing in their professions so they wanted to stay where their jobs positioned them and not be transferred.

I got my elder orders in 1978!

I've been an elder for forty-five years and am still preaching, teaching, and serving the Sacraments.

Today, over 50 percent of the people attending seminaries in the United Methodist denomination are women. In the almost fifty years since my ordination, more women are answering God's call than ever before and becoming ordained!

Many people have called me a "pioneer," but I'd rather think of myself as a person wrestling with the medical ethical issues of my era that will extend to many generations beyond me, perhaps my great-great-great-grandchildren.

I rather doubt that Dr. J. knew about my "beginnings" in the ministry. But he must've approved of women in the ministry; otherwise, why would he give me his beloved crucifix?

I don't believe that Dr. J. knew about my United Methodist ordinations and dilemmas concerning the denomination's questions about being transferred from one church to another.

Did it matter to him that I am a Protestant, and he was a Catholic? Why would he give me his crucifix, the symbol of the Catholic Church, whereas the symbol of my Protestant church is a cross?

=========================================

20

# Chapter 3
## Cross-Crucifix

Cross and crucifix are two words that are often confused.

Crosses are found in most Protestant churches and are meant to remind the believer of the sacrifice that Jesus made for the salvation of the world through his suffering and resurrection. The word *cross* is derived from the Latin word *crux*, meaning the stake upon which criminals were hung. The plural form of cross is crosses. The symbol of the cross is mostly favored by Protestant religions.

A crucifix is an artistic rendering of a cross with the body of Jesus depicted on it. A crucifix always depicts a corpus on the cross. The crucifix is mostly used as a Christian symbol in the Catholic Church.

For thousands of years, Christian art has depicted Christ crucified or Jesus on the cross at Golgotha. Such a depiction of the death of Jesus shows Him wearing a crown of thorns, with a sign inscribed "INRI," which stands for Jesus of Nazareth, King of the Jews.

The word *crucifix* is derived from the Latin phrase *cruci fixus*, which means one who is affixed to the cross.

The crucifix is Good Friday, and the cross is Easter Sunday. Both have their merits. Both are powerful symbols of the Christian faith.

An interesting question was asked of the God Squad concerning the crucifix and the cross. *The God Squad* was an American television program featuring a Roman Catholic priest and a rabbi who answered questions asked by the audiences.

One of the questions was "Is it proper for a Methodist to wear a crucifix that was given to them from a family member who died?" The answer was "Accepting the crucifix was clearly an act of love but wearing it might create confusion. There's no canon law prohibiting non-Catholic Christians from wearing a crucifix, but wearing one commonly indicates that you are Catholic."

By contrast, Protestants wear crosses, without the body of the crucified Jesus. The crucifix focuses on the crucifixion of Jesus as his primary gift. The empty cross focuses on the resurrection of Christ.

Christ's suffering and dying for the sins of the world are present in their most searing and inspiring form in the crucifix. However, Christianity also focuses on the resurrection, which reminds Christians that the man who died on the cross was not a man at all but God.

================================================

**Regardless, Dr. J. gifted me with his crucifix, even though I am a Protestant and a woman. I'm not sure if he knew how often I visited Roman Catholic churches after I realized my United Methodist religion endorsed the woman's right to choose to have an abortion. Obviously, my newfound prolife ethics didn't fit with my religious affiliation of Methodism. So, I started attending local Catholic churches to seek out their sanctity of life views. It wasn't long before I recognized that only men were allowed to become priests.**

**Women did not have a place of authority as clergy in the Roman Catholic doctrine. People would say to me,**

"Women aren't in the ordained ministry. Why would you, a woman, want to be ordained? Jesus only called men."

Fortunately, I completed my Biblical research on this issue, and I could rightfully claim Jesus treated all people equally and called all of us to "follow Him."

Yet, it was difficult to be a prolife United Methodist clergywoman. I simply didn't fit in with the teachings of the United Methodist Church, and I certainly couldn't become a Roman Catholic clergy, because they don't allow women to become priests.

When I was a chaplain at Wilmington General Hospital, there was an incidence where I served a Roman Catholic female patient Holy Communion, and after she received the elements, she looked at me and said, "You're a woman!"

I said, "Yes," whereupon she immediately spit out the wafer (body of Christ) and grape juice (blood of Christ) and screamed, "I can't take communion from you. You're a woman. I'll burn in hell for that!"

Apparently, the hospital's unit clerk had given me the list of Roman Catholic patients who wanted Communion, instead of the Protestant list.

It wasn't long after I felt redeemed when our hospital administrator called me at home begging me to please hurry back to the hospital. It seems a large group of nomad travelers had erected tents on the grounds of the Wilmington General Hospital because their leader was a patient on the oncology floor, and they didn't want to leave her.

Their leader was a female who was considered the figurehead in their community. The nomad travelers were grieving the cancer that had metastasized into their leader's liver and pancreas.

In all, there were eighty-two men, women, and children who participated in the lawn sit-down and wouldn't leave the hospital grounds.

My hospital administrator met me at the hospital and exclaimed his dismay at all their people in the hospital room too. In all, there were twenty-two people gathered in and outside her hospital room.

"It's against the *rules*! Get them out of here! They're a menace and won't listen to me! Get them off our hospital grounds, and only two allowed in her room at a time!" exclaimed the hot-headed administrator.

When I approached them, as the hospital chaplain, I explained that only two people were allowed in her room at a time and asked them to please clean up the tents all over the hospital grounds.

They huddled together and then pronounced they would listen to me because I was a woman, and this group of nomad travelers honored women. They removed their tents, took turns visiting their sick female leader, and welcomed my prayers and presence that I shared with them until their leader died.

The nomad travelers had listened to me and followed my suggestions.

I finally found a place where I was accepted as a clergywoman!

Whenever I need to feel God wants me to be a clergywoman, I reflect to the day I needed to buy my first robe to officiate at my first funeral.

The service was for a forty-six-year-old man, my dad's age when he died. I'd become quite close to their family, his wife and three children, as they reminded me of my family. They asked me to wear a clergy robe for his funeral, and I had no idea where to get one, as all the robes back then, were tailored for men's sizes. Cokesbury is the United Methodist store for books, clothing, and all kinds of clerical needs.

When I entered the Cokesbury store, I felt strange asking for a woman's clergy robe. The salesman told me they didn't have any women's robes, but he had a small-sized men's robe that had just been returned, so the price had been reduced.

When I put the robe on, a chill went through me, as it fit perfectly.

"I'll take it," I exclaimed proudly.

"That'll be $128.50," he said with authority.

"Okay," I said as I reached into my purse and brought out our checkbook. No Visa/MasterCard in those days.

As I was writing the check, I realized I didn't have sufficient funds in the bank to cover the cost of my new robe. But I wrote the check anyway, the first time I'd ever done anything like that without conferring with my beloved husband.

As I drove back to Wilmington, Delaware, I wondered how I was going to admit this lack of judgment to my husband, who is financially disciplined.

"Hi, honey," I sheepishly murmured, ready to step up and tell the truth about the check and robe.

Tom said, "Hey, don't forget we're going to my Rotary party at the Brandywine Race Track tonight. It starts with a five thirty buffet, then the races follow."

Oh dear, when am I going to tell him about the overdraft? We'll need to do something soon, or else the check will bounce!

We had already asked our eldest daughter, sixteen-year-old Debbie, to babysit her sisters, thirteen-year-old Becky and our youngest, eight-year-old Carrie.

I stuffed my newly purchased robe in the hall closet, out of sight, and then we went to the harness racetrack, the first and last time I've ever attended.

I didn't know how to choose horses then or now, but my Tom asked if I wanted to bet on the "daily double."

"What's that?"

"It's when you choose two horses to win, one in the first race and one in the second race."

Without thinking, two numbers immediately came to mind. "I'll bet on number 5 and number 3," I responded, not registering why I chose those numbers.

"Why those horses? What are their names?" he inquired.

"I don't know."

So, Tom dutifully put two dollars on number 5 for the first race and number 3 for the second race.

Obviously they won, or I wouldn't be telling this story, but the irony is that the win of the daily double was $128.50, the *exact* price of my new clergy robe I had purchased a few hours earlier.

Tom, who's seldom impressed, excitedly asked me why I chose number 5 and 3?

"I have something to tell you, honey. Today, I bought a clergy robe and it cost $128.50, and I remembered on the back of the robe's collar are the *numbers 5 and 3.* I put the robe in our hall closet at home."

To prove myself, I asked Tom to call our daughter Debbie, so she would look in the closet, open the zippered robe, and find the back collar of the robe.

"Yes, Dad, there are numbers 5 and 3 on the back of a black robe. Why? What's going on?" she queried.

"Nothing, just checking."

None of the Rotarians knew I was going to seminary or anything about the robe, but they knew I won the daily double, and all of them asked me, "Who are you going to bet on for the next races?"

I didn't bet a penny after that and haven't bet on horses since, but you can bet I put that $128.50 in the bank the next morning to cover the check for my new clergy robe.

Not only that, but I couldn't tell anyone about how I got that money at the racetrack, because the

Peninsula-Delaware Methodist denomination had a stringent, rigorous policy against gambling at that time.

Interestingly, the United Methodist other social policy agreed on a woman's "choice of terminating her pregnancy with an abortion," but you couldn't bet on anything.

What a dichotomy!

===================================

# Chapter 4
## When Is a Person a Person?

When I began my ministry, it was because of the Delaware abortion law that would allow women to have an abortion if the embryo would cause "undue emotional stress to the physical or mental health of the mother, or substantial risk of the birth of the child with grave and permanent physical deformity or mental disability."

That was Friday, June 13, 1969.

Since that time, the US Supreme Court on January 22, 1973, *Roe v. Wade*, declared "a pregnant woman is entitled to have an abortion until the end of the first trimester of pregnancy without any interference by the state."

Each state was then allowed to determine "when" they would allow a legal abortion. Some states, such as Delaware, do not have a time period on "when in the nine-month pregnancy there would be a time an abortion could not be surgically done."

Since that time, God only knows how many babies in the first trimester, second trimester, and last trimester have been destroyed.

The question is "When is a person a person and protected by the Constitution?" A right to an abortion can't be found in the Constitution of our country. The Supreme Court could not find nor has it found a way to describe when a person is a person and therefore protected. With the fetus's status as a human being in limbo, the most the court would say was that fetuses beyond the thirty-eighth week have "potential life." A curious phrase, inasmuch as some fetuses (babies) of even lesser age have survived outside the womb.

Miraculously, some have survived despite efforts to abort them.

The first such case in our State of Delaware was at the Wilmington Medical Center hospital where I was a chaplain. It was reported in the *Morning News Journal* on June 7, 1979, "two infants were born alive following saline abortions."

The salt solution injected into the mother's womb usually kills the fetus. However, two nurses detected a pulse in the umbilical cord and immediate life-support measures were taken."

The two nurses who found those infants had me paged, and I went to the area where they rescued those two children. I'm forever grateful the babies were resuscitated and later adopted by caring people.

In fact, there are other people who have survived abortions, and they've formed a group entitled, "Abortion Survival Network."

This organization's website has an informational page that reads,

> Although the exact number of abortion survivors is unknown, even the exact number of abortions completed annually even in the United States is incomplete, (as states like California do not report the statistics and the number of chemical abortions across the country are not reported), what we have found

is that there are far more abortion survivors than most people would suspect. Although many abortion survivors were subjected to late term abortion procedures, there are children who survive abortion procedures in first and early second trimester abortions, including chemical abortions. With the assistance of the abortion pill reversal, we now see children surviving due to this intervention. From 2012–2020, the Abortion Survivors Network had contact with 336 survivors of abortion and their friends or family who contacts us on their behalf. Interestingly enough, a pro-life writer estimated that based on the failure rates of late-term abortions, there could be as many as 44,000 survivors of late-term abortion in the United States alone. It's important to note that although our culture often talks about late-term abortion being rare, the reality is that there are a significant number of late-term abortions that occur.

The founder of the organization is Melissa Ohden, who was fourteen years old when she learned that she was a survivor of a botched abortion. Melissa lives to tell her personal story of love and redemption as she searches for and finds her birth mother.

Her intensely personal story of love and redemption illuminates the powerful bond between mother and child that can overcome all odds. Her book is entitled *You Carried Me.*

When is a person a person? Ask those survivors of abortions.

Another life-saving not-for-profit prolife organization is Skylark, which provides resources for women and men who are facing issues with unplanned pregnancies. They offer free pregnancy tests, ultrasounds, parenting classes, maternity clothes, and baby items. As an affiliate of Care Net, Skylark utilizes an effective educational tool—the Compassion, Hope, and Help Training Curriculum. Their private BYD (before you decide on an abortion) eleven-week sessions include the decision-making process, life skills, foster families, adoption, and even linking each person with a nondenominational church family close to their residence. No one is alone because Skylark volunteers' primary purpose is to bond with each person who comes to them needing guidance concerning their unplanned pregnancy. They've served 22,500 women and men since 1992 with 947 babies saved, thanks to their president, Patrick Eades, and his team.

I delivered a prayer for the unborn at the New York Right to Life convention in 1979 and was asked to repeat my remarks at other Right to Life conventions.

My remarks were as follows:

> At this New York Right to Life Convention
> with special remembrance of the International
> Year of the Child, I bring news from the State
> of Delaware.

This summer, at our medical center, two tiny infants were born alive even though they had saline abortion procedures. One weighed two pounds four ounces, a boy. The other, a girl, three pounds, four ounces. These two babies survived insurmountable difficulties. However, two alert nurses, who cared about whether the babies lived, took the little ones and placed them in the premature nursery.

What have we heard about saline abortions?

We've heard it said that saline abortions would result in rapid deaths for the baby, but that isn't true. The babies lived for many hours before they were discovered.

We've also heard it said that saline-aborted babies would have permanent brain damage, but that isn't true. These babies, after two months in our ICU nursery, have tested perfectly normal. We've heard it said, these would be "unwanted" babies, but that isn't true, the babies have been easily adopted.

To these two babies and many millions of unborn children, I dedicate this prayer today:

O God, we come to you today in the midst of all kinds of death.

There is death in the air we call ... smog.

There is death in the water we call ... pollution.

There is death in the cities we call ... racism.

There is death in infanticide we call …
alleviating suffering.

There is death in euthanasia we call …
mercy.

There is death in suicide we call … one's
own right.

O God, we come asking for life: new life for
ourselves, for all people, for our world. Make
us aware of your presence and power, God.

Come like a breath of fresh air.

Come like a drink of clear water.

Come like the embrace of another person.

Come like protection in the womb.

Come like compassion for a helpless infant.
Come like reverence for all life, as you make
no distinction between quality or non-quality,
more precious or less precious.

We thank You, Lord, for this company of
caring friends.

We ask that whatever else is said about us,
it will be said that in the midst of death, we
brought life to the unborn, to the sick and
maimed, and to all life. We brought Your love.

Amen.

==========================================

**Did Dr. J. hear this prayer somewhere in the Right to Life
groups he might've attended? Did he attend any Right to
Life groups?**

**I wonder these thoughts every time I write something that Dr. J. could've read or heard.**

**Why did he give me his crucifix? What did he know about me that would've promoted a gift so precious? I'm going through my journey looking for Dr. J.**

==========================================

What has been happening in the field of medical ethics since the abortion ruling on January 22, 1973?

*Roe v. Wade* has brought forth forty-eight years of controversies.

The most recent arise from congressional attempts to reverse or modify the decision. *Roe v. Wade* boils down to this: a woman has a constitutionally protected right to seek an abortion. It is an absolute right during the first three months of pregnancy. After that and up to the point of viability, which the court defined as the capacity of meaningful life, the right may be limited only by the state's interests in protecting the health of the mother.

After viability, which the court reckoned to occur at the seventh month of pregnancy, the right may be limited and even proscribed by the state's interest in "the potentiality of human life, unless abortion is necessary to preserve the life or health of the woman."

A wide range of scholars holding both pro and antiabortion beliefs quickly pointed out the numerous problems with *Roe v. Wade*. These included mistakes in history, science, and law, but the essential difficulty was, as it remains today, that *Roe v. Wade* imposes on the nation a view of the abortion issues lacking constitutional warrant.

What should our courts of law do? When does a person have a right to be protected by the Fourteenth Amendment? The Fourteenth Amendment to the US Constitution was adopted on July 9, 1868, as one of the Reconstruction Amendments. The amendment, particularly its first section, is one of the most litigated parts of the Constitution, forming the basis for landmark decisions such as *Roe v. Wade* (1973). The amendment's first section includes several clauses: the Citizenship Clause, Privileges, Due Process Clause, and Equal Protection Clause. The Citizenship Clause provides a broad definition of citizenship, overruling the Supreme Court's decision in *Dred Scott v. Sandford* (1857), which held that Americans descended from African slaves could not be citizens of the United States. The Due Process Clause prohibits state and local government officials from depriving persons of life, liberty, or property without legislative authorization.

When is a person a person with inalienable rights?

There have been two Supreme Court cases in our country that have attempted to identify personhood.

One was written in 1857: *Dred Scott v. Sandford* was a landmark decision by the US Supreme Court in which the court held that African Americans, whether slave or free, could not be American citizens and therefore had no standing to sue in federal territories. In this case, Dred Scott attempted to sue for his freedom. In a seven-to-two decision, the court denied Scott's request.

In the second Supreme Court case, *Roe v. Wade*, the court ruled that a right to privacy under the due process clause of the Fourteenth Amendment extended to a woman's decision to have an abortion but that this right must be balanced against the state's two legitimate interests in regulating abortions: protecting prenatal life and protecting women's health. The Roe decision defined "viable" as being "potentially able to live outside the mother's womb, albeit with artificial aid," adding that "viability" is usually placed at about "seven months (twenty-eight weeks) but may occur earlier, even at twenty-four weeks."

Here are the similarities of those two US Supreme Court decisions on slavery and abortion:

*Slavery* 1857
Although she or he may have a heart and a brain and may be a human life biologically, a *slave* is not a legal person; the Dred Scott decision by the US Supreme Court has made it clear.

*Abortion* 1973
Although he or she may have a heart and brain and may be a human life biologically, an *unborn baby* is not a legal person, according to the *Roe v. Wade* decision by the US Supreme Court.

---

*Slavery* 1857
A black man or woman becomes a legal person when he or she is set free. Before that, he or she has no legal rights.

*Abortion* 1973
A baby only becomes a legal person when he or she is born. Before that, she or he has no legal rights.

---

*Slavery* 1857

If you think that slavery is wrong, then nobody is forcing you to be a slave owner, but don't impose your morality on somebody else.

*Abortion* 1973

If you think abortion is wrong, then nobody is forcing you to have one. But don't impose your morality on somebody else.

---

*Slavery* 1857

A man has a right to do what he wants with his own property.

*Abortion* 1973

A woman has a right to do what she wants with her own body.

---

*Slavery* 1857

Isn't slavery really something merciful? Every black man has the right to be protected. Isn't it better never to be set free than to be sent unprepared and ill-equipped into a cruel world?

*Abortion* 1973

Isn't abortion really something merciful? Every baby has a right to be wanted. Isn't it better never to be born than to be sent alone and unloved into a cruel world?

---

Fortunately, in 1868, the Fourteenth Amendment overturned the Dred Scott decision by granting citizenship to all those born in the United States, regardless of color.

Let's hope and pray reversing the *Roe v. Wade* decision will grant citizenship to all persons who are formed at conception. However, knowing how the Dred Scott case and the Fourteenth Amendment have not really changed the negative attitudes about our Afro-American brothers and sisters, even 150 years later, I don't expect the baby in utero has much of a chance either.

Most states do not have a law to protect the baby in utero. The potential mother can have an abortion even in the third trimester, the last three months of pregnancy.

Why would they be born alive? Because late-term abortion procedures performed on fetuses means that the baby cannot easily be lifted out of the womb. They are too large.

As we know from many abortion survivors, the saline solution often doesn't work. The other second trimester abortion technique, a surgical opening of the womb through a small abdominal incision to remove the fetus has a much higher incidence of live fetuses.

At what point does the fetus (baby) have rights?

Again we need to ask, "When is a person a person?"

There have been hundreds of court cases concerning late-month abortions throughout these years.

One of the most infamous was Dr. William Waddell in California. Dr. Waddell was brought to trial by two nurses who testified that he not only ordered them to not help resuscitate a two-pound-twelve-ounce baby girl born following a saline abortion, but Dr. Waddell was seen actively strangling the aborted baby.

Testimony in both trials indicated that the baby girl had survived the abortion performed on her seventeen-year-old mother, she was alive in the newborn nursery, and she had a good chance of surviving as a normal child. Both juries did not convict the physician. They asked the question for which there is still no answer even though it's been deliberated by many juries all these years.

The jury asked, "How could it be all right for Dr. Waddell to kill the baby on the morning of March 2 while still in the womb of her mother but murder if he killed the same baby several hours later in the newborn nursery?"

In another case, Dr. Kermit Gosnell was charged with killing infants who had survived abortions. He even trained his employees to use surgical scissors to sever the newborn's spinal cords just below the base of the skull.

Although Gosnell referred to these practices as "snipping," the word doesn't convey the nature of the act. Even though there were a dozen eyewitness testimonies and tiny bodies recovered from the freezer at Gosnell's "house of horrors" abortion clinic, the judge dismissed the murder charges against Gosnell for the deaths of three of those infants.

The news was shocking. How could anybody fail to see the abundance of evidence that these infants had been born, had struggled to live, and had been murdered? These cases point dramatically to the unresolved legal, medical, and moral dilemmas in our abortion practices.

This practice is called "infanticide."

There are many books about infanticide and personhood. When, indeed, is a person a person?

The book *Indicators of Humanhood: A Tentative Profile of Man*, written by Joseph Fletcher, a theologian and professor of medical ethics, has proposed a set of "positive human criteria" specifically designed to serve as indicators of "personhood" in decisions regarding abortion and infanticide. Dr. Fletcher was pro-abortion, pro-infanticide, and pro-doctor-assisted-suicide. He wrote the following criteria of when a person is really a person.

Dr. Fletcher advocates to be called "a person," that "person" must have the following:

1. Minimal intelligence: below 40 on the Stanford-Benet is questionably a person, below 20 not a person.
2. Self-control. If the condition cannot be rectified medically, a person without control is not a person.
3. Capability to relate to others: this includes both interindividual and diffuse social relationships. If not able to relate, the individual is not a person.
4. A person must have a control of existence: when absent leads to state of irresponsibility.
5. Balance of rationality and feeling: a person can be neither coldly rational nor given over completely to feelings. If he or she is, the individual is not a person.
6. A person must have a sense of time: a sense of the passage of time. If not, he or she is not a person.
7. A person must have a sense of futurity, a sense of time to come, looking forward, and planning. If not, he or she is not a person.

8. A person must have a concern for others. If not, he or she is not a person.
9. A completely isolated individual who cannot communicate, as opposed to being disinclined to communicate, is not a person.
10. A person must have neocortical function. If not, he or she is not a person.

Should these be the ways to define when a person is a person?

How is infanticide defined? It is allowing babies to die.

Should we save our defective infants, or shall we allow infanticide?

In an article from *Fidelity* magazine written by James Bruen Jr., this is his commentary: "Abortion may be the silent holocaust, but it is not invisible. Newspapers advertise its availability; feminists tout its necessity; politicians genuflect before this 'reproductive right,' and pro-lifers' express outrage over its legality. Infanticide, however, is almost invisible."

There was one case that brought a lot of attention in the media. Baby Jane Doe was born with spina bifida, that is the failure of the spine to close properly, and hydrocephalus, excess fluid on the brain.

The first neurologist who examined her recommended the usual treatment for babies in her condition: surgery to close the spinal opening and inserting a shunt in her head. The parents consented, and the baby was transferred to the hospital for surgery. However, the parents then heeded the advice of another physician who recommended no surgery.

What should our courts do? Should the family accept the child? Or does the disabled child have a right to life? The courts could find no answer.

When is a person a person?

As Dr. Seuss said in his *Horton Hears a Who* book, "A person is a person no matter how small."

When does science say human life begins?

Dr. Robert George wrote the following in his book titled *The Embryo*:

> Human embryos, whether they are formed by fertilization, natural or in vitro, or by successful somatic-cell transfer (cloning), do have the internal resources and active disposition to develop themselves to the mature stage of a human organism, requiring only a suitable environment and nutrition. In fact, scientists distinguish embryos from other cells or clusters of cells precisely by their self-directed integral functioning. Thus, human embryos are what the embryology textbooks say that they are, namely, human organism-living individuals of the human species—at the earliest development stage."

Science has clearly and decidedly proven that a new human life begins at conception, the moment sperm and ovum meet and form an entirely new self-directing living organism of the human species with its own individual DNA distinct from both mother and father.

The procedure to discover if your "baby" in utero is deformed is called amniocentesis. It's a procedure in which amniotic fluid is removed from the uterus for testing or treatment. Amniotic fluid is the fluid that surrounds and protects a baby during pregnancy. This fluid contains fetal cells and various chemicals produced by the baby. Amniocentesis is performed to look for certain types of birth defects, such as Down syndrome, sickle cell, cystic fibrosis, muscular dystrophy, Tay-Sachs, and similar diseases. Because ultrasound is performed at the time of amniocentesis, it may detect birth defects that are not detected by amniocentesis, such as cleft palate, cleft lip, club foot, or heart defects.

There are some birth defects, however, that will not be detected by either amniocentesis or ultrasound. If you are having an amniocentesis, you may ask to find out the baby's sex. Amniocentesis is the most accurate way to determine the baby's gender before birth.

Does amniocentesis mean you'll abort the baby if he or she is found to have an anomaly? What would you do if your amniocentesis found your baby had a disability?

If you're a parent, do you remember when you found out you were pregnant? The first question from others usually was, "What do you want, a boy or a girl?"

And the answer usually was "I don't care as long as it's normal."

Most families want children who are "normal," that is, without disabilities. If you know you're going to have a special needs baby, often abortion is chosen.

After all, don't you want to preserve your right to ensure

that no one with disabilities will be born into your family? The abortion debate is not just about a woman's right to choose whether to have a baby. It's also about a woman's right to choose which baby she wants to have.

It sounds logical, doesn't it? Does she want a disabled child? How about the father, does he want to pay for and care for a special needs baby?

What would a disabled child bring to the family except a lot more effort, more expenses, more suffering that they would have to endure?

Many argue, "It's my choice to not want a disabled baby. It's my choice to abort. You can choose to have a deformed child, but I don't want one." Does the disabled child have any rights at all? When should he or she have his or her right to be called a person?

======================================

I wonder, would Dr. J. think a disabled person is a person with his or her own rights? He was a pediatrician and devoted his life to taking care of all children, regardless their infirmities. He must have believed in the sanctity of life, over and against the quality of life. In fact, my dissertation for my Doctor of Ministry degree from Palmer Seminary is entitled "An Experimental Study of the Impact of a Program on the Medical Options of Sanctity or Quality of Life upon Nursing Students." The purpose of that study was to design an ethics course, eleven weeks long, that employed both sanctity-of-life and quality-of-life approaches. The ethics course I developed was to determine whether the course of instruction would aid students to clarify their own attitudes and value preferences concerning quality and sanctity of life. The adaptations for the course came from a variety of sources, but they were assembled specifically for the ethical dilemmas of abortion, euthanasia, infanticide, and suicide.

Did Dr. J. believe in the sanctity of life?

I'm still searching, trying to remember if Dr. J. could've known about my working with disabled children.

How did Dr. J. feel about these children? He must've had an opinion.

Oh, how I wish he would've talked with me about his innermost thoughts concerning the disabled child.

=======================================

# Chapter 5
## The Disabled

Years ago, because of my involvement with special needs kids, I was invited to speak at the Annual Handicapped Person award luncheon. The use of the term *handicapped* was accepted some years ago. Recently, "handicapped" has been replaced with the use of the word *disabled*, as referring to people with disabilities.

It was there Walt Huntley presented me with this poem that I've saved through the years.

God's Hall of Fame
This crowd on earth, they soon forget
when you're not at the top
They'll cheer like mad until you fall
and then their praise will stop.
Not God, He never does forget,
and in his hall of fame
I'd rather be an unknown here
and have my name up there.

---

All of us have genetic defects. All of us have handicaps. Who will decide which to eliminate? Do the disabled have a right to live?

If so, what is meant by the word *live*?

Does it refer to mere survival or to a quality of life? What does it do to people when they must struggle each and every day to overcome barriers?

What is the answer, and how do we find it? Is the issue one of money and priorities, ethics and charity, politics and power, attitudes and feelings, rights and wrongs, bricks and mortar, or science and technology? Who will make the recommendations, and who will decide?

The barriers confronting disabled people are immense, but there is one central problem that seems to underlie most of these obstacles, and that is the problem of right. Rather than asking the question, do I have a right to die, what the disabled people most desire is the right to live. They desire only what is available to Americans who are not disabled. The requests are for the simple right to life, to learn, to work, to determine their own goals and lifestyle, to earn the respect of others, to obtain housing, to secure transportation, to receive needed treatment, to enjoy cultural and entertainment offerings.

What barriers have we built around our disabled? As might be expected with a group as large as sixty-one million adults and over three million children under the age of eighteen who are disabled Americans, of course their needs, desires, and problems vary widely. There are, nonetheless, some central issues common to the group as a whole.

There are architectural barriers. For example, deaf persons cannot hear spoken announcements or auditory-based warning signals, so it would help to print instructions in lights that would be accessible to them.

Elevator buttons typically are placed above the reach of people in wheelchairs.

Ramps enabling people in wheelchairs to circumvent stairs are often sloped too steeply, presenting dangerous obstacles, while inclined ramps may provide no resting spots for wheelchairs.

There are educational barriers. Of the estimated three million disabled youth, fewer than half are receiving an appropriate education. Even more basic is the entire question of segregation of children by their disabilities rather than by their abilities and interests. Education and careers for the disabled in the mainstream of American life remain more a goal than a reality.

Few are tested for their abilities but rather are measured in terms of their disabilities. Would you like someone to only look at your infirmity, instead of your God-given potentials and strengths?

Also, there are legal barriers for the disabled. They have faced employment discrimination and had many of their rights taken from them but were not given their inalienable right: their right to life.

Sometimes insensitivity threatens the lives of disabled people. Persons with disabilities are especially vulnerable to crime, because they present inviting targets to muggers, rapists, vandals, and other criminals. Blind pedestrians cannot see their assailants, deaf shoppers cannot hear them, and paraplegic individuals cannot flee.

Each one of us has a disability. What is yours? Perhaps it isn't physical but attitudinal. Is our attitude one of being fearful? Attitudes toward disability are often negative because we fear disabilities that we don't understand, and we feel uncomfortable in situations where we experience fear and uncertainty. Yet these problems can be overcome. Fear can be put aside by offering information that makes disabilities comprehensive, and uncertainties can be reduced by helping people understand how to be with those who are disabled.

Better attitudes will happen when the average citizen looks at a woman in a wheelchair, a man with a hearing aid, or a child with crutches not as people who can't but as people who can. We must learn to see the person behind the chrome wires, the wooden cane, and the spiked wheels.

What is your disability?

For one person, it may be the habit of self-indulgence and for another, a fear-bound look on life, being afraid to try anything new. For someone else, the disability might be a vile temper. For another, it may be laziness; another may suffer with compulsive eating, drinking, gambling, or drug abuse.

Perhaps your disability is an emotional one, a broken marriage, a painful onslaught of arthritis, so that you can no longer hold a tennis racket, let alone a golf club. It could be a sudden change in health, and you find yourself facing a long-term illness, or your malady may be a bitter disappointment in business.

It is not easy to experience any one of these or a dozen situations that do happen throughout our lives.

Those who are unprepared for the problems they will face throughout their lives are not really conditioned for life.

The high rate of emotional illness and the incidents of drug abuse, alcoholism, and suicide are evidence that people have trained for success and perfection when they ought to have trained for failure, the failure of preparing oneself for the probability of problems and infirmities.

Some years ago, a friend was going down a ski slope, in high hopes for another thrilling ride. Instead, she got a concussion, internal injuries, and a hospital bed. Something happened on the way down. She hit a tree.

Since then, she's been a student in the university of pain, multiple operations, and periodic hospitalizations. Her own preferred plans have been disrupted.

Somewhere along the road, we all must deal with disabilities in some form of disrupted plans, deferred hopes, and unrealized dreams.

Wallace Hamilton had this one-liner in his book *Ride the Wild Horses*: "every person's life is a diary in which they mean to write one story and end up writing another."

It has been suggested more than once that life makes progress in a resisting medium. The bird needs the resistance of the air to fly. The fish needs the resistance of water to get traction for its fins. We would not be able to stand up without the resisting action of the law of gravity. Sometimes the weight of life keeps us going.

We can learn from others who are disabled.

From the deaf, I have learned a sensitivity to loneliness. I have learned to touch and smile and communicate without clever subtleties.

The mentally disabled have taught me that concentrating on my climb to the top of the ladder of success only decreases my ability to enjoy simple trust and honesty in relationships.

What do the physically disabled teach me? Those with cerebral palsy have taught me that the quality of life has nothing to do with physical ability or attractiveness. Through them, I have learned to communicate with and value a friend's spirit.

Blind friends have taught me the joy of trust and closeness that can occur when one is willing to risk dependence on another.

From the mentally ill, I have seen my own vulnerability and need for love. I have learned to value hope and celebrate growth and change.

From the health impaired, I have learned of a spiritual strength that can grow through suffering. Grieving and suffering can bring me closer to God, if I allow my feelings to embrace that thought.

My perspective has changed.

I have come to believe that the most handicapped are those of us who measure human value by physical beauty and the ability to compete with charm and wit.

Sharing life with a handicapped friend forces me into finding that essence of life that is deeper and more lasting than superficial appearances.

Every one of us has a handicap to overcome.

I have mine; you have yours.

Judging your disability as better or worse than mine only sets us over-against one another. You're not running my race, and I'm not wearing your track shoes.

We're really competing with ourselves.

Every disability offers that same alternative: either it dominates you, or you are dominating it. A corollary is that once a disability has been dominated, it ceases to be a disability but becomes an asset.

How do we accept other people and ourselves with our own peculiar disorders?

Hear this plea from one of my special needs friends:

### Blessed Are You

Blessed are you who talk to the deaf in moments of quiet silent love.

Blessed are you who hold our hand in the darkness never pushing your light but allow us to hold our own.

Blessed are you who take time to listen to slower speech, for you help us to know that if we persevere, we can be understood.

Blessed are you who walk with us in public places and ignore the stares of strangers: for in your companionship, we find havens of relaxation.

Blessed are you who never bid us hurry up: and more blessed are you who do not snatch our tasks from our hands to do them for us: for often we need time rather than help.

Blessed are you who stand beside us as we enter new and untried ventures: for our failures will be outweighed by the time when we surprise ourselves and you.

Blessed are you when by all these things you assure us, the thing that makes us individuals is not in our peculiar muscles, not in our wounded nervous systems, but in

the God-given self which no infirmity can
confine.
Rejoice and be exceedingly glad and know
that you give us assurances that could never
be spoken in words.

---

Thank you, dear friend Bessie, who was born with cerebral
palsy and lived eighty years with a severe disability. She
lived a full life and communicated with those willing to be
patient with her slower speech.

Handicaps, disabilities—we all have them.

===============================================

Now I am wondering if Dr. J. knew of my participation with
the disabled, as I was on the Easter Seals, American Red
Cross, and United Way Boards of Directors. In all these
community outreaches, I volunteered in their special
needs for children and adult programs.

I am so deeply appreciative of Dr. J's thoughtful,
heartfelt gift of the crucifix. I'm still searching through
the last forty years of my life trying to discover how he
could've known me.

Perhaps my crucifix-giving pediatrician friend, Dr. J.,
heard my sentiments about the disabled people. After all,
his obituary said, "his interests also included the early
recognition of mental, physical and genetic developments
of children." Although I don't remember seeing him in
any of the places I spoke, still he could've read about my
involvements.

Even though it was possible, I don't believe Dr. J. was

in Legislative Hall when the first abortion law was passed in 1969. And I'm unsure of whether he was connected to any infanticide issue. However, I do believe he's an antiabortion, pro-life because Dr. J.'s obituary said he was a member of St. Mary Magdalene Catholic Church.

Every one of my Roman Catholic friends that I've met through the Right to Life group are prolife and antiabortion.

In fact, the catechism of the Roman Catholic Church states, "Since the first century the Church has affirmed the moral evil of every procured abortion. This teaching has not changed and remains unchangeable. Direct abortion that is to say, abortion willed either as an end to a means, is gravely contrary to the moral law" (No. 2271).

According to George Weigel, a biographer of John Paul II, "Any serious understanding of Catholic social teaching begins with the dignity of the human person from conception until natural death. That is the fundamental principle: to claim that you are thinking within the social doctrine of the church and to support abortion on demand or euthanasia is simply wrong, it's a logical fallacy."

In our society today, there are many who profess their religion as Roman Catholic but still believe abortions are a choice.

I'm always amazed when top-ranking officials of our country are Roman Catholic, yet they endorse abortions and in some cases even infanticide and euthanasia.

I'm dismayed they've abandoned their religious teaching yet still pretend to be Roman Catholic.

====================================

# Chapter 6
## The Good Death

What does "the good death" have to do with Dr. J. and why he would give me his family crucifix?

Only because I'm still trying to discover where he might have met and known me well enough to give me something so personal and precious.

Perhaps I met Dr. J. at the Wilmington Medical Center, Delaware division.

Now I'm back to the beginning of my journey when I visited EBTS Seminary and Dr. Maring encouraged me to be the first woman to be enrolled in the Master of Divinity program. However, Tom's and my savings accounts were being held for our children's future education. I wanted to sign up for the Master of Divinity degree, but we certainly couldn't pay for ninety-six hours, the length of time to procure a degree at any seminary.

Then, two days later, in the *Wilmington News Journal*, an ad said, "Come hear Dr. Joseph Fletcher, writer, author, lecturer, on 'Euthanasia. The Good Death.' All are invited to the Wilmington Medical Center."

How interesting because I'd just finished reading another one of Dr. Fletcher's books. This one was called *Situational Ethics*, where he proclaimed, "in the matter of voluntary passive euthanasia, we must learn to walk before we can run. The question of who shall speak for those who are incompetent or incapable of speaking for themselves must wait until the general public *accepts the fact that abortion or the killing of live cells is permissible.*" Then he continues his rhapsody by saying, "there are more Typhoid Mary's carrying genetic diseases than infectious diseases. We have an 'obligation' to prevent the birth of genetically diseased or defective children."

And then, *"popular attention centers on the abortion movement at the other end of life, euthanasia is concerned with the responsible termination of life. The more we can relate these two movements practically the better, because they are both concerned with the responsible care of human life, one at the beginning and the other at its end"* (my emphasis).

Remember, Dr. Joseph Fletcher also wrote about infanticide in his book *Tentative Profile of Man*, where he identifies the 10 indicators of when a person is a person.

I always believed the act of abortion would lead to the act of euthanasia and infanticide, as you're actively taking the life of someone else.

So, I was anxious to attend Dr. Joseph Fletcher's lecture on "Euthanasia, The Good Death."

Educational and informational it was, indeed.

It changed my life as much as the Delaware Senate Bill Number 200 that allowed abortions for women "who would be emotionally and mentally disturbed if they had a handicapped embryo."

At the lecture, Dr. Fletcher, world-renowned author on medical ethics, preached the importance of dying a "good death." "Too much money is spent on the last months of life when the person is dying anyway, why keep them alive?" he boldly claimed.

Dr. Fletcher's presentation was eloquent, even convincing the likes of me to temporarily agree with him.

Somehow, I found my voice and with great gusto said, "Why don't we allow everyone over the age of seventy-two to have a choice of living or dying? Perhaps give them a 'hemlock pill' in case they choose death. Of course, it would be their choice," I sarcastically implored.

And then, I snidely added, remembering Delaware's original abortion bill, "Of course it would be with the approval of two doctors, one psychiatrist and the other a medical doctor."

I was sadly surprised when so many people who attended the lecture turned, looked at me, and then applauded. Was it possible that people would choose a hemlock pill if they were ill?

After the lecture with Dr. Fletcher, I walked up to speak with him, as I was trying to understand a man of his intellect promoting such an antilife position.

It was then I met the chaplain of the Wilmington Medical Center. He was so pleased I spoke about giving people hemlock pills because, as a chaplain, he had witnessed everything wrong about the medical system. "They continue hooking people up on machines and giving them chemo when their veins collapsed and stints became infected," he boastfully proclaimed. "We should give them a pill and let them die."

He misjudged me, thinking I actually approved giving people the "good death" hemlock pill.

The chaplain then talked about needing someone to help him visit patients at the Wilmington General Hospital, better known as the Alpha/Omega Hospital. This hospital was a place where most babies were born, and most people died. During the years from 1960 to 1980, there was a large oncology unit at the General Hospital where most cancers were treated, and many patients stayed until they died.

The chaplain continued, "We really need some volunteers at the Wilmington General Hospital."

I knew I had no choice. I blurted out, "I've been to Eastern Baptist Theological Seminary two days ago and might be taking classes there. Maybe I can help."

The chaplain immediately replied, "No kidding! I'm a graduate of EBTS, and if you volunteer at the General Hospital, our chaplain's office could pay for your seminary classes and books in exchange for visiting patients."

Are you kidding me?

I rushed home and told my husband, "I've got my books and classes paid for."

Tom, shocked, uttered, "At what price?" He was referring to the time I wouldn't be home to cook meals and be the "normal" mom I had been for the past sixteen years.

The following day, I drove up to EBTS and signed up for one class, "The History of Christianity," given by Dr. Norman Maring.

It was early September, and I was volunteering at the General Division three days a week, two days at seminary, and I didn't have a clue how I was going to study after all these years or speak to dying and sick patients and their families.

I ended up studying with our daughters, as there was a small area right off their bedrooms. Fortunately, they didn't mind my presence in their private boudoirs and even volunteered to help fix breakfast when I had an 8:00 a.m. class and prepare dinners when I came home late.

I thanked God daily for our three daughters, who were willing to help when I needed them.

At my seminary, one of the courses was "Field Education." Many of the hopeful seminarians chose to be serving in a church as an assistant to fulfill their field education obligation.

I was assigned as "health-care chaplain" at the Wilmington General Hospital, and that chaplaincy lasted the entire eight years I attended seminary with my Master of Divinity degree and two more years as I graduated with my Doctor of Ministry degree.

==================================================

**I could've known Dr. J. when I was the chaplain, but he was a pediatrician with his own practice, and sick babies were patients at another hospital, the Delaware Division of the Medical Center.**

**Could Dr. J. have been at Dr. Joseph Fletcher's meeting and heard me herald the hemlock pill? I doubt it because, as time passed, I became an advocate against giving the hemlock pill and doctor-assisted suicide. And I fought against expanding living wills, which Dr. J's wife, Iris, a Delaware politician, later introduced in the House of Representatives.**

==================================================

Reflecting back to Dr. Joseph Fletcher's lecture on "The Good Death," remember that he advocated for the right of every patient to choose when he or she wanted to die.

Should we allow people to choose when they want euthanasia? Should someone be designated to assist in a suicide? Who decides that a patient is, indeed, terminal? Let's define the words *terminal* and *euthanasia*.

An article entitled "Terminal Is for Buses, Not Patients," written by Justin Stein MD, it states,

> "It is very distressing to hear about reports on the management of cancer patients with terminal disease. The use of the words, "terminal cancer," does great disservice to patients and the medical profession. I am reminded of Dante's Inferno, "abandon hopes all ye who enter here!" The word "terminal" signifies the abandonment of hope. We should not revert to the days when there were hospitals for the incurable. The word "terminal" should not be used by oncologists. If a physician who is treating a patient with cancer takes away all vestiges of hope, there is very little left for the patient."

The history of euthanasia goes back to ancient times. The first recorded use of the word *euthanasia* was by Suetonius, a Roman historian, in his *De Vita Caesar um-Dives Augustus*, to describe the death of Augustus Caesar.

> Augustus's death, while termed "a euthanasia" was not hastened by the actions of any other person. Withdrawal or with holding treatment

60

was practiced in history, the correct term for this is *orthothanasis* which means "passive death." In this method, the actions of curing the patient are never applied and his death is made easy in a passive form.

There are four different classifications of euthanasia. They are:

1. Voluntary passive involves a person who dies with his or her consent.
2. Involuntary passive involves a person permitted to die without his or her consent.
3. Voluntary active involves a person's death at his or her will, with doctor-assisted suicide.
4. Involuntary active involves a person being killed without knowledge or consent.

The first objection to euthanasia came from the Hippocratic oath, which says, "I will not administer poison to anyone when asked to do so, nor suggest such a course." But according to the NOVA "The Hippocratic Oath Today" article by Peter Tyson, "today most graduating medical school students swear to some form of the oath, usually a modernized version. Only 9% of modern oaths prohibit euthanasia."

So, with the Hippocratic oath out of practice, where is the opposition to "administering poison" to anyone when asked to do so or suggesting such a course?

It's difficult to oppose a person's right to self-determination concerning decisions about treatment.

However, if our society decides that it's a person's right to his or her own body, then we need to see these decisions may fail to consider that a significant fraction of patients pronounced terminally ill by their attending physicians survive for a much longer period than predicted.

Also, with the rapid advance in medical science, today's "extraordinary" measures may become tomorrow's standard procedures. Importantly, extraordinary measures may make a terminal illness less painful and distressing.

There are times that tube feedings, chemotherapy, and radiation therapy might prolong life and are purposeful, allowing the patient to die without enduring the pain of bed sores, which relate to malnutrition, a by-product of withdrawing water and food from the patient.

What are the criteria for defining when a person is not a person anymore but a dead person?

Back in the eighteenth century, one way of determining if a person died was to hold a mirror, soap bubbles, feather, or candle to the nose to detect respiration. In the nineteenth century, death was determined by the lack of a heartbeat.

Fortunately, some tepid soul decided to beat on the heart with what we now call CPR and brought some "dead" people back to life. Thanks to modern technology, we can now transplant hearts and other organs.

When you look at how the definition of death has changed through the centuries, you realize how far medicine and science have evolved, changing the definition from "holding a mirror under the nose to flat electrocardiogram

(EKG, which checks the rhythm of your heartbeat) to a flat electroencephalogram (EEG, which indicates an irreversible coma)."

It's obvious the definition of death is impossible to determine. Each generation of scientists, doctors, and willing patients who undergo difficult procedures will bring a new definition of when a person is dead.

When is a person a person?

=============================================

**I wonder if Dr. J. ever wondered about that. When is a person a person? He must've thought about it when he encountered abnormal and handicapped children in his practice.**

**As he aged and became sick, he might've thought about his illness and what would become of him. After all, he thought about his family heirloom, the crucifix, wondering what he should do with it.**

**Why and how did he choose me to treasure such a keepsake?**

**Would he favor "the good death"? Did he know how I felt about euthanasia and death and dying?**

=============================================

# Chapter 7
## Death and Dying

Death.

No one wants to talk about it.

At least no one did when I was a chaplain at the hospital many years ago.

Now people talk about it openly, without borders.

I'm frankly glad that as a society we're talking about death as though it was real, honest, and true, which it is.

Early on, I learned an important lesson when I was a "chaplain-in-training," at a hospital in Philadelphia, Pennsylvania.

Part of becoming a hospital chaplain meant that I had to observe a "teaching" chaplain as we went on rounds together, much as doctors do training their interns. I, along with four other wannabes, would move from one patient's room to another asking them questions and trying to determine their needs.

As we entered one room, the teaching chaplain advised, "This patient is in a coma, and she hasn't woken up from her last alcoholic binge."

After the chaplain spoke, the so-called comatose patient abruptly sat up in her bed and loudly proclaimed, "I was not a drunk!" and then zoomed back into her comatose position.

I thought perhaps the chaplain had the wrong room. But the chaplain fainted, and we all ran for the nurse. Apparently, the comatose patient had been in that state for six weeks. I don't know when or if she died, as the teaching chaplain never answered questions about her whereabouts.

My lesson learned. Patients can hear people in the room. Don't speak derogatorily.

Never, never speak out loud in front of the patients about anything you don't want them to know or hear, even if they seem to be comatose.

And another important fact I learned was that patients can wake up after being comatose.

Doctors had little hope that Munira Abdulla would ever wake up after suffering a brain injury in a 1991 car crash in Mainz, Germany. She woke up twenty-seven years later.

In a two-part series on *The Early Show*, national correspondent Tracy Smith tells the story of Sarah Scantlin, a woman who woke up from her coma state after twenty years. After two decades of floating somewhere between life and death, Sarah Scantlin is fully and finally awoken.

There are so many lessons to be learned in life and in dying. Yes, we are all going to die someday. As the old saying goes, there're two things that we'll have to do in life. Pay taxes and die. Some folks don't pay taxes, so there's truly only one thing we'll have to do in life. Die.

My first encounter with a dying patient was with the Wilmington Medical Center's chaplain as he was guiding me around to visit hospital patients. The patient was elderly, comatose, and hooked up to some strange-looking machines.

The chaplain, right in front of the patient, said, "Marlene, this is the kind of person Dr. Joseph Fletcher was talking about. She would be dead, if not for all these contraptions hanging off her already dead body."

A chill went through me. Why did I feel such compassion for this poor soul who probably would be better off dead and living in heaven? I didn't understand my deep anger at the chaplain for saying what was obvious to everyone but me: "She would be better off dead."

My field education health medical chaplain position was undefined, so I could walk around, see patients, and talk with families, nursing staff, and everyone in the hospital.

I didn't know where to start, so I just went from room to room, especially in the oncology (cancer) unit.

In the 1970s, patients usually died in the hospital, especially if you had a "tumor" or a "lump."

No one called it the "C" word—*cancer*. However, most every patient I visited knew they had the Big C and asked me if their family members knew that they knew.

I didn't know.

Family members would ask me, the chaplain, "Do they know I know that they have it? How can I talk with them? What do I say?"

That's how the support groups started.

Orderlies helped me gather the patients together in the common room, and we talked about their feelings, their fears, their fear of dying. They especially wanted their loved ones to know they knew.

So, I formed another support group. This one was for families of the patients. We would meet once a week and talk about their fears, their hopes, their concerns about their loved ones dying.

Then I assembled the group of patients and their families, and they would finally talk about what they should've been talking about throughout their loved one's illness.

Talking about your feelings, getting them out in the open, sharing with family and friends are vital to your mental, emotional, and consequently your physical well-being.

Little by little, family members would tell their story about their loved one. As I started to know the patients and their families, I realized we all have similar fears, hopes, angers, loves, and rainbow of emotions. We are complicated people, even when our lives are riding the waves gently.

During my early days at the medical center, I was fortunate to encounter Dr. Elizabeth Kubler Ross, who'd just written a book entitled *Death and Dying*. She became an instant best-selling author and traveled around the world identifying the stages of death and dying.

I became personally involved because I volunteered our family home to be her residence while she was lecturing at a variety of forums.

It was during that time I listened to and talked with many cancer patients, with Elizabeth guiding me on my new journey.

When Elizabeth's mother died in Switzerland while she was visiting our home in Delaware, that solidified our relationship, and we continued corresponding through the years.

I quickly learned Elizabeth's identification of the five stages of dying the patient and the family will experience.

Denial, isolation, bargaining, and anger are usually prevalent with each patient and his or her family, but the most difficult stage is acceptance. If members of a family can share these emotions together, they will gradually face the reality of impending separation and come to an understanding and acceptance.

The most heartbreaking time for the family is the final phase, when their loved ones are slowly detaching themselves from their worlds, including their family.

Probably the most arduous time for everyone concerned is the moment the patient's mind slips off into a dreamless state, the need for food becomes minimal, and the awareness of the environment all but disappears into darkness.

This is a rough period for the family members, as they aren't sure whether to stay or leave. "How long before death takes place?" they frequently asked.

Many are afraid to leave their loved one for even a bathroom break.

I would recommend to families to eat properly and try to get some rest.

This is the time when families need help the most. It is the time for the therapy of silence with the patient.

It is hard to die, and it will always be so, even when we have learned to accept death as an integral part of life, because dying means giving up life on this earth.

But if we can learn to view death from a different perspective, to reintroduce it into our lives so that it comes not as a dreaded stranger but as an expected companion to our life, then we can also learn to live our lives with meaning and full appreciation of our definiteness of the limits on our time here on earth.

Then how do we live with the word *death*?

As a hospital chaplain at the Wilmington General Division, I encountered death almost daily.

It wasn't long before I was asked to officiate at funeral and memorial services for the oncology patients I visited. It was an honor to be invited to participate in these services, because it helped family members find some closure. However, I found that loved ones need a lot more than just the memorial service.

After the funeral, after the relatives have gone back to work, after the neighbors have stopped coming by, so often, the house seems too still, the bed too big, and the feelings of grief too complex, unspeakable, and precious to bear alone or even to share. But if they are not shared, especially by the widow or widower, they can become a fierce wall of loneliness.

Realizing all these feelings that death brings to the grieving people, I started a support group I entitled You Are Not Alone.

A Roman Catholic priest friend, Father Bill Keech, and I were in a number of clergy meetings, and we talked frequently about the abortion issue. Soon we realized our deep concerns for the widows and widowers who felt so alone in this couple world of ours. Of course, my mom becoming a widow at the tender young age of forty-four made me realize how lonely life can be for a widow.

I asked Father Keech to help me cofacilitate the group, and we met at the American Red Cross building in Wilmington. We were there every Friday from 1:00 to 3:00 p.m. for ten years.

The You Are Not Alone group helped me understand

pain, loneliness, and suffering, as I vicariously lived my life through their difficult journeys.

Death.

For me, it was knowing I would be "graduating," as Rev. Dr. Roy Burkhart, the minister of my youthful years, proclaimed.

We're just moving on into another realm with God as our guide and His Son, Jesus the Christ, as our Lord and Savior.

In the meantime, we must learn how to grieve our losses.

===================================

**Did Dr. J. believe this too? I don't think he ever attended any of my lectures on death and dying or visited my church when I was preaching about any of these issues. Did Dr. J. ever send anyone to the support groups?**

**I do wish I could've talked with him and heard his thoughts concerning children and death too. Surely, as a pediatrician, he experienced a lot of death surrounding children, as I was encountering too.**

===================================

# Chapter 8
## Death of a Child

Our daughter and son-in-law, Becky and Bud, recently lost their precious daughter, Megan, who, at the tender age of thirty-three was tragically struck by a car while riding her bicycle preparing for a triathlon event. Her sudden death is a tremendous loss to our entire family and for all who knew our outgoing, assiduous, caring granddaughter.

There is nothing right or good or bearable about the death of a child. It seems morally wrong to have life taken away, almost before it has been lived, but one of the facts of life is that death comes to all ages.

Contact with a dying child and his or her family can strain the emotions of everyone.

At the Wilmington General Hospital (WGH) where I was the chaplain, my first encounter with a child dying was at birth. Most births in the State of Delaware, at that time, were at the WGH, and as the health-care professionals got to know and trust me, they called about newborns who were born dead. I was amazed, in this medically efficient world, how many women delivered a stillborn. I didn't know what to say to the distraught families who were expecting a birth, only to have something medically turn sour and the baby suddenly be born dead.

The first time I was paged to aid the mother, father, and family members who had a stillborn, I blundered through, saying a prayer for its soul and pretending to understand. After I finished, the mother turned to me and sadly pronounced, "You didn't mention my baby's name!"

I hadn't even thought about that. Of course, they'd picked out a name. What was the matter with me that I was so out of touch? And I was a mother too. How would I have felt if one of our three daughters had been a stillborn?

After that experience, I wrote a graveside homily for every child who died at birth. And, importantly, if the family approved, I baptized every one of them. The baptism became crucial because the grieving families had a piece of paper with their child's name on it.

Remember, there's no birth certificate, because the baby wasn't born.

There's also no death certificate, because the baby didn't die because it wasn't born.

But now there's a baptismal certificate indicating the child was a person.

Every family who had a stillborn baby really appreciated this acknowledgment of their named child who never had a chance to live outside the womb, even though the families had prepared for nine months in hopeful expectation of a live birth. It was a sad, difficult time, as are miscarriages.

I had already started the You Are Not Alone support group and two-family support groups in the oncology unit of the hospital, so I started another support group. I named it *HOPING* (Helping Other Parents in Normal Grieving). We met in the chapel of the Wilmington General Hospital once a week.

This started with families who had a stillborn, and then many parents who'd lost their baby to accidents, crib deaths, and disease began coming to the support group.

As I listened to the emotions expressed by the caring

family members, I learned a lot about their feelings and concerns.

I jotted down some of their comments:

"I'm numb, from my toes to my head, and I can hardly breathe at night, much less sleep."

"I've become a person I don't know and don't want to know. I'm scared."

"Should we have another child?"

"I just don't want to go on. There are times when I'm feeling suspended."

"There's this hopeful mother right up to a quarter to twelve and at one twenty-five, boom. My child is dead! There is no such thing as forgetting."

"We go to the cemetery all the time. I think about all the changes I'm going through, and I can't get myself together for anything."

"I feel like screaming a lot of times. I feel like getting into my car and just going, where I don't know, just to go and get away."

"I'd rather have a devil on earth than an angel in heaven."

"I'll tell you one thing: I'm scared to even let my other children go out of the house."

"I've wanted to die. I have really wanted to die, because so much of me has been buried."

"There were times when I felt anger and disbelief, and then one day I thought to myself, all I have are some clothes and a crib. Maybe God has something better. I don't know."

These are just some of the comments I heard as the facilitator of the *HOPING* support group. The group provided a setting for sharing all experiences and feelings.

Supportive feelings come from knowing that all the group members have undergone a similar and profound emotional experience. The need to share, if only in silence, is important.

Losing a child is devastating. There's no time period that will ease the family's pain from this loss. The memories parents have of their child prior to his or her death and while she or he is dying are very poignant, vivid, and enduring. To give up the memories is to give up the child.

Parents need to ruminate about the past.

I've seen many couples struggling to stay together after the loss of their child, because everyone grieves differently. It's vital to understand and sympathize with your spouse's different grieving process. Each person grieves in his or her own individual way. There is no "right" way or "wrong" way of grieving.

However, the more parents share their bereavement, the better it is for all concerned.

As I was new at this facilitating, I asked the support group members of You Are Not Alone and HOPING whether the group helped them or not.

Here are some of their comments:

"I found it helps a lot to share my experience; that's why I keep coming back to the meetings."

"Sharing here together is so important. But even more important is giving support to each other."

"Well, I certainly learned we've all experienced the same agony."

"After six months our relatives had their own lives again;

that's why the group, with all of us going through the same anguish, helps me grieve."

"To the parent, anger, sadness, misery, despondency just doesn't go away. It keeps popping right back in there. You need someone who's gone through what you're going through to talk to."

"Even if I go to a meeting, and don't open my mouth, it's nice being in the room with people who have gone through this sorrowful trauma."

"I was desperate. I went through the whole thing for months. You get to the point where you feel guilty letting your friends know this, because you don't want them to say to you, "Maybe you should go and see somebody.""

As I facilitated the support groups, I discovered that they provided a setting for sharing any and all experiences and feelings of those who attended.

The group, with its support, serves as a vehicle for sharing and attenuating the sense of isolation. The parents feel they are not alone even though there are no immediate answers to the loss of their child. However, as they share a common experience, the blow is softened, the pain diminishes, and they gradually integrate the event into their life experience.

======================================

**Did Dr. J. know about these support groups and perhaps send any of his patients' families to participate?**

**It wasn't long before our HOPING support group reached out to local pediatricians and other medical personnel, and I spoke to their groups. However, I don't**

remember Dr. J. inquiring about the group. Nor did I hear his name, supporting our support group.

During this time period, another dilemma presented itself. An excellent physical therapist at the Wilmington General Hospital was fired after twenty-four years of service, the last four years as chairman of the Department of Physical Therapy. He came to my office in despair because he was abruptly dismissed five months before his twenty-fifth year, which would've given him a lot more earned pension money. Immediately I went to the hospital administrator and asked, "Why?" I was told it was none of my business; they could do what they pleased. I presented this dilemma to my two volunteers, Mildred Bromwell and Drew Patterson, and together we decided to resign in protest. Four months after I resigned, the following article appeared in the Wilmington News Journal:

"Ex-Chaplain at Hospital Takes City Church Post

> The Rev. Dr. Marlene Walters, the hospital Chaplain who resigned in June to protest the personnel policies at the Wilmington General Hospital, has been appointed Associate Pastor at Grace United Methodist Church. She will be performing general pastoral work including Support Groups, and visitation. Dr. Walters earned a Doctor of Ministry in medical ethics from Eastern Baptist Theological Seminary. She resigned from the chaplaincy when Sidney L. Raymond chief physical therapist at the General Division was abruptly dismissed after more than twenty-four years of service at the medical center. Since then, personnel policies at the medical center have been changed so that top officials will now

review any proposed terminations of senior staffers."

Of course, I was pleased the Wilmington General Hospital changed their policy, and I was proud to support the members of staff who had worked all their lives just to be terminated close to retirement. Now, at least, "top officials will review any proposed terminations of senior staffers."

I'm beginning to wonder if Dr. J. knew about Wilmington Medical Center's errant firing policy. Did he know Sid Raymond, the one I defended? It's certainly possible because Sid worked with young children as well as adults.

Perhaps that's why Dr. J. gave me his treasured heirloom, the crucifix.

=====================================

# Chapter 9
## Grief Recovery Group

The decision to resign in protest was very difficult. I really liked my position at the Wilmington Medical Center, and as I reflect on those days, depression was part of my new idle life.

The last time I was that depressed was when my precious dad died suddenly ten days after Tom, and I were married. We were on our honeymoon in Florida only to be called back to Columbus, Ohio, because my loving father had a brain aneurysm that suddenly, sadly, took his life.

I can totally relate with people who are depressed and unhappy. I went through a lot of depression after my dad died, and now I was going through grief and depression again. I really missed my chaplaincy appointment and friends at the Wilmington General Hospital.

My dearly beloved husband, Tom, in order to renew my interest in gardening had a half-ton truck full of mulch delivered to our back door. The idea was for me to "get back to work, do something useful." I appreciated his effort, but the idea of doing anything was overwhelming. I was depressed. I had no energy. I lost my concentration. I lost my usefulness. I was lost.

After we resigned, my friends became my new support group, especially Mildred and Drew, who had volunteered with me at the General Division.

And people from the support groups I started would call and express their feelings in support of my decision.

Four months later, Grace United Methodist Church offered me an associate pastor position in their city church. I was pleased because they wanted me to continue my support groups.

Grace Church owned a facility called Charis (Grace) House. The lovely home was unused, and it was adjacent to the Methodist Country Home, a place for senior citizens. It was at the Charis House that I facilitated the HOPING support group and a new group for children who'd lost a loved one.

Losing a child is very difficult, and now, people in the community were asking me about how to handle their children's grieving of a parent's, grandparent's, or friend's death? How do we help our children grieve?

So, I started another support group called Grief Recovery Group (GRG). This support group was for families to bring their children so they could grieve together as they recovered the loss of their loved one.

I had no idea how to facilitate such a group, nor did I have anyone who was willing to cofacilitate any of the groups, but I realized most grief-stricken people just need someone to listen and care. I did care, and I was willing to listen.

Now, I was into another phase of my learning curve, and I put together some thoughts about what we need to remember about children's grieving the death of a loved one.

The basic issue is not *whether* to talk to the child about his or her serious concerns but *how* to talk to him or her. In order to help children, cope with the problems of death, it is necessary to develop an environment in which they feel perfectly safe to ask any questions and are completely confident of receiving an honest answer.

Many parents wanted me to speak to their children alone, in the safe environment of the Charis House.

Years before I went into the ministry, I was a member of the Junior League of Wilmington and became a puppeteer, as our group went to elementary schools to present different programs.

We wrote a script surrounding the issues of death and dying, so when I met with the children to explain what dying meant, I used a lot of those scenarios and even had the two puppets I made from my Junior League days.

It's amazing how each child would look directly at the puppet, knowing it was connected to my arm and speak frankly, openly telling the puppet his or her problem. My two puppets' names were "Salty," a dog puppet, and "Harvey," a bunny puppet. I used each puppet on my two arms and tried to change my voice pitches to have Salty and Harvey sound different, but I was not a ventriloquist.

===========================================

**Would it be possible that Dr. J. heard about Salty and Harvey? I rather doubt it; however, our Junior League group of volunteers went to many schools and performed for the children. Dr. J. was a leading pediatrician in the State of Delaware and might have heard about these programs.**

**Perhaps he knew about Charis House at Grace United Methodist Church and the grief recovery support group.**

**Or he could've listened to one of my lectures at**

different schools, hospital seminars, symposiums, and conferences, explaining the lessons I learned about children's grieving.

===================================

# Chapter 10
## Children's Grieving: Lessons I Learned

As I began to communicate with young children, I was discovering the variety of emotions they embraced.

Children are acutely attuned to the wavelengths of their environment. Consequently, when a child's environment signals that certain subjects are not to be discussed, being too painful for the adult to death with, children can become mute, outwardly accepting the adult's benign words of falsehood but inwardly feeling abandoned.

Consequently, the little ones are left to cope with the fears and anxieties by themselves, at the very time they need to seek all the strength and support available. When the channels of meaningful communication between the child and the adult become blocked, the youngster must go elsewhere for answers. Depending on the age of the child, anger toward self is not uncommon.

When other people in the family are discussing the loss of the loved one, your child immediately knows that there's something very serious because his or her entire surroundings change. He or she quickly senses that the people whom they trust and love are now keeping something from them, something frightening. It is as if the environment had said, "Please don't ask me about this because it is too terrible."

If the death is yet to occur, all the family should talk freely to one another. Open discussions of the problem can do much to mobilize family strength.

Many children believe firmly that the death of their loved

one is punishment for their misbehavior. The mother who warns her child, "It's raining; you'd better wear your boots, or you'll get sick and land in the hospital," cannot even imagine how sharply those words are recalled when, two weeks later, he or she lands in the hospital. The illness may be unrelated to that rainy morning when the child chose to disobey, but in the child's eyes, there is a connection.

This is also true of the child who wishes harm, as all children do at some time or another, to their brother, sister, mother, or father.

In the children's heart of hearts, they know that someone is punishing them for their wicked thoughts, and they can easily translate those thoughts into feeling guilty.

As a hospital chaplain, I always wanted the entire family to visit their dying loved ones in the hospital. At first, I worried that the children would accidentally trip over an IV tube or grab the needle that connected grandma's vein to the intravenous bag hanging over the bed. Many worries entered my mind, but children have a unique understanding of dread and almost always enter the hospital room with a sense of heart-loving compassion.

The very first family I invited to visit their dying loved one entered the room with a rambunctious five-year-old yelling, "Nana! Nana!" As she ran to the bed to embrace her nana, I could only project the damage she was going to do pulling out the IVs from the wrist of her beloved grandmother. I needed not worry. The child stopped short of grabbing her nana's wrist and said, "Oh, Nana. You have a boo-boo. Let me kiss it." Then, thoughtfully, she kissed her nana's bandage-free elbow.

When a child encounters death, whether it is through losing a relative, a friend, a pet, or only through hearing a reference to death in a television show, it is no longer possible to spare that young one of the word *death*, no matter how young the child might be. Their curiosity has been stimulated; as with every new experience the youth have had, they will want to know more about what they've discovered.

To thwart such natural, healthy curiosity in a youngster can have very unhealthy effects on their emotional development.

One of the worst effects is the selective shutting off curiosity limited to those things in the world that, like death, cause painful emotional responses. The children perceive that, although their parents eagerly encourage their wishes to know about many pleasant things in the world, they divert the children's curiosity away from unpleasant things, particularly something as unpleasant as death.

Children sense, through cues from their parents, that death causes extremely painful feelings inside people.

The young ones then further observe that their parents try to avoid the inner painful feelings by withdrawing all their attention from the offending point in the outside world, such as the concept of death, and the youngsters are bound to join forces with them in their ostrich policy. Like the ostrich who hides his head in the sand in a vain effort to do away with a real danger, the children withdraw their attention and curiosity from death in order to deny that it really exists.

In doing so, the children's ultimate purpose is to protect

themselves from the painful emotions that the concept of death might produce.

If the young ones don't know what death is, then they don't have to feel any of the anxiety or sadness or even anger that contemplation of a loss through death always causes.

Some people in the support group wondered what harm there is in allowing or even encouraging a young child to develop an ostrich policy toward something as disturbing as death.

If it were merely a matter of postponing a piece of learning about the world the child lives in, the danger might not be as great, but the postponement is based on the erroneous premise that a young child must be shielded from any knowledge about the world that will cause him or her painful emotions. Feelings like sadness, anxiety, or anger get pushed inside, as the youngsters develop an ostrich-like defense mechanism, burying their thoughts about any situation that could evoke such dangerous feelings.

As a result, those children suffer a double limitation upon their lives. In the outside world, they can only permit themselves to know about things that do not cause painful feelings. In their inner world, they will inhibit all painful emotions.

To be deprived of access to painful emotions is not an asset; it is a serious liability. To touch a hot stove but to feel no physical pain can lead to a serious burn because there was no signal to withdraw from the dangerous heat.

To face a dangerous situation but to feel no anxiety may lead to an inappropriate response.

To experience a loss through death but to feel no sadness

is to be deprived of the most helpful signals a person can have to stimulate the necessary mental reactions to adjust to the loss.

Children who do not learn to permit themselves such appropriate emotional distress are in danger of growing up to be shallow people, cut off from a normal depth of human feeling and lacking emotional responses to life.

Just as young children need help in learning about the outer world, so will they need help in learning about their inner world of feelings.

It may seem paradoxical that children must be taught about something already inside themselves, but not everything inside is known in their sphere of conscious attention.

In order to accomplish a greater understanding of what is perceived, grown-ups need to help their children become better acquainted with the outer world by teaching them words they can use to name things. I found that assigning words to children's feelings further helps them to be fully conscious to what they feel, so that they are unlikely to inhibit feelings by such techniques as the ostrich policy.

*Do*

- call out your crying as the sadness you feel.
- call out your anger as anger that you feel.
- call out your feelings and show you love and care for them no matter what they feel.

Still another way children are helped to cope with their own feelings is by giving them an opportunity to observe how grown-ups handle their feelings. If, in explaining sad feelings due to death, a grown-up shows a child her or his own sensitivity through appropriate words and behavior, this, in time, helps the youngster comprehend the unpleasant and unfamiliar emotions he or she is feeling.

Here are some of the basic thoughts I've learned about children who are grieving.

1. Children will almost always remember a loss, even if they don't talk about it, they will remember. Even if they were too young, they will remember images and feelings.
2. Children cannot and should not be protected from emotional pain. Often adults want to protect themselves through their children. Children know what is happening. Allow them to share their feelings with you.
3. Children experience the same losses as adults. Don't assume that a parent's loss won't affect his or her children.
4. Parents may not always be aware of losses in their children's lives (for example, a pet in school, a friend's grandparent). Take time to talk and listen to your child.
5. Children are capable of grieving.
6. Children understand loss, death, and finality in age-appropriate ways.
7. Helping children with grief involves more than confronting the child with reality. Patience, understanding, love, and support are needed as well.

8. There is no right or wrong way to grieve. Children grieve differently than adults. They may express less sadness, talk less, and cry less. This doesn't mean that they aren't grieving. They're just doing it their own way.

9. One parent cannot make up for the loss of the other parent. One person cannot be two. Most children understand this.

10. If a child's grief wasn't addressed at the time of the loss, there is always a second chance, and a third, and a fourth, no matter how old the child is.

11. Grief-work is not always a time of devastating sadness and tears. There are moments of sweetness, as members of the family remember the joyous moments of life.

12. Grief-work is an opportunity for growth, a time for finding new strengths and sharing feelings with those we love.

13. Avoid making hasty decisions or major changes in your life too soon. The family needs the security of old memories, and time may alter your viewpoint.

14. Try to be flexible about demands on yourself and your children; difficult times call for modifying your standards.

15. Don't expect too much of yourselves or your children at times of crisis. Nonessentials can be delayed.

So, how do we help our children through this grieving process?

Grief is an extremely difficult and engaging process. A

grieving person must focus on him or herself during this period, and rightly so. Many times, however, we overlook the fact that grief comes in all sizes and ages. Therefore, children are often ignored during mourning, with the rationale that, "they wouldn't understand."

The grieving process in children is highly complex, since so much depends upon each child's stage of development. For instance, a three-year-old's understanding of death and the mourning process will be quite different from that of a ten-year-old.

Both would be very different from a sixteen-year-old. Yet, there are many fundamental similarities between a child's grief and the adult mourning process. It is important to understand that grief work provides vast potentials of growth for all ages.

The following is a list of suggestions for helping your child through the grief process:

- Set a time aside to talk with your child. Explain the events occurring, why you are crying and sad.
- Use basic words, like *die* and *dead* to convey the message.
- Use the deceased person's name when referring to him or her.
- Avoid the phrases that soften the blow, such as "sleeping," "went on vacation," and "God took them." This will only confuse and scare your child.
- Let your child ask questions and answer truthfully. Be honest, simple, and direct. If you don't understand something, let your child know that, too.

- Be sensitive to the age of your child and her or his level of understanding. Don't offer information beyond the child's comprehension, as it will only confuse matters.
- Tell stories that will increase your child's awareness.
- Read or have your child read children's books related to death.
- Play with your child. Use puppets, drawings, dolls, or toy soldiers. Play in ways that will allow the child to express his or her feelings.
- Watch for TV programs that might help your child's understanding.
- Talk about God with your child. Pray with your child.
- Share your feelings and experiences with the child.
- Let your child participate in what he or she wants to—visitation at the hospital, going to the funeral, visiting the cemetery. It is very important that you don't pressure your child into doing any of these things but allow him or her to be involved if he or she wants to.
- Accept help from others to watch your children and talk with them, but remember, you are the most important person to your child.
- You are a role model for your child. If you hide your grief, your child will learn the ostrich policy too.
- We should understand our own grieving process, since these things are communicated to the child.
- Let your child vent his or her emotions and acknowledge them.

- When approaching the problem, break it down into manageable pieces rather than an overwhelming whole.
- Watch for telltale signs of maladjustment, such as eating or sleeping or depression disturbances over a period of time.
- Seek pastoral or family counseling if the grief is unresolved.
- Watch for earlier mourning experiences of your child. For example, a child often experiences death for the first time when a pet dies.
- Remember a child will have the same feelings we have but a different level of understanding.
- Communicate your appreciation of having the deceased person around.
- Discuss and have your child recognize changes in routine due to the death.
- Plan something that you and your child can look forward to.
- This is perhaps the most important of all. Please do not be disappointed or angry if your child does not understand or appreciate the death. He or she is going through a learning experience and discovery. Give him or her time!

The experience of dying is a normal life stress, with which all human beings must cope as they grow, mature, age, and die. There are certain common normal reactions to the natural experience of dying.

Children who are six years old or younger have no

clear concept of the finality of death. Young children do know that people die, but in their minds, death happens to other people. Death comes with a boom or a splash and is something done to someone by someone else. Children of these ages do not have the emotional ability to visualize themselves as old, nor do they anticipate injury or accident. They usually feel completely protected by their parents, their teachers, and the police.

When the five-year-old little boy says to his mommy, in a fit of anger, "I wish you were dead." What he is really saying is "I wish you would go away, perhaps next door, but not so far away that I cannot call you back when I want you."

Death to young children is completely reversible. Any suggestion that dying may mean a personal total separation is immediately and anxiously denied.

The actor in television is shot dead one day but then appears hale and hearty on another program the next day. Though squirrels lie dead by the roadside, identical squirrels are actively bouncing around the nearby trees. Pets die and are missed, with sadness, but frequently immediately replaced.

Children ages seven to eleven begin to appreciate the emotional significance of personal death. Normal denial defenses are quickly established to minimize anxiety, but additional emotional reactions specific to this age group will complicate helping.

When a sympathetic adult tells a bereaved child that the deceased parent or grandparent is happy up there in heaven with God, the child may react with anger at being abandoned.

Children will wonder why Mommy or Daddy decided to leave and may even suspect, with a feeling of guilt, that their own naughtiness was responsible for the departure of the parent. It is more helpful to your child to tell him or her that the parent did not really want to leave but was so sick that God brought the parent to be with Him in heaven.

If you don't believe in heaven, then tell your child what you believe, even if you explain that you're not sure, but you will always love him or her.

When schoolmates go to the hospital and never come back, a grade-school child misses his or her friends but considers them to be out there in some vague hospital. The fears of the child about death and dying may be focused on a phobic reaction to hospital or treatment institutions.

The child's specific reaction to the prospect of death is the emotional response to the threat of separation, the fear of not being with Mommy or Daddy.

The grade-school child begins to realize that when friends or grandparents die, they are seen no more. Your child knows that means the removal and loss of loved ones. When Mommy dies, the anguished normal reaction of the grade-school child is "Why did Mommy leave me?"

To the young grade-school child, death represents a separation but still a continuation of physical existence. In death, your child anticipates the person dying will be joining Aunt "Nelle" up there in heaven. But heaven in the hereafter still has the emotional significance of being just around the next block.

It is a separation and a loss but not really the end of the physical existence. Although this separation anxiety may be too frightening to be openly admitted, the separation, loneliness, and terror may heighten the child's fears of isolation.

Every child should be reassured that he or she will never be left completely alone and will never be abandoned.

=====================================

**Did Dr. J. teach the children in his practice how to grieve? Did he ever come to one of my lectures about children and death? I've searched around to see if he's ever written anything about children and grieving. I will continue to look, but I'm sure Dr. J. believed all children should be reassured they would never be left alone or abandoned.**

=====================================

One of the mothers of the Grief Recovery Group gave me these remarkable stanzas of poetry that underlines what our children need from their parents, teachers, and family members.

# Children Learn What They Live

## by Dorothy Law Nolte

If children live with criticism,
they learn to condemn.
If children live with shame,
they learn to feel guilty.
If children live with tolerance,
they learn to be patient.
If children live with encouragement,
they learn confidence.
If children live with fairness,
they learn justice.
If children live with security,
they learn to have faith.
If children live with approval,
they learn to like themselves.
If children live with acceptance
and friendship, they learn to
find love in the world.

# Chapter 11

## Families of Suicide to Enable Recovery (FOSTER), Youth Suicide Prevention Program (YSPP), Adult Depression Group (ADG), and Supporting KIDDS (Kids Involved in Death, Divorce, and Separation)

After I had spent three years as associate pastor at Grace United Methodist Church, the bishop and cabinet appointed me to Mt. Lebanon United Methodist Church. I finally had my own church, even though Mt. Lebanon's membership had dwindled to fifteen active members. So my new appointment would be for just one year to celebrate Mt. Lebanon's sesquicentennial, and then I would get another appointment.

Mt. Lebanon's fifteen members were pleased we would be using their small but available rooms for our support groups.

Many of the people who attended the Grief Recovery Group were recovering from their loved ones who committed suicide. They asked if I would start a support group specifically for families whose loved ones had committed suicide. It became obvious that people who were grieving the loss of someone from a natural death are much different from those who's loved one committed suicide.

I named the new group Families of Suicide to Enable Recovery (FOSTER). I was surprised at how many people came to this group, bringing their entire family and supportive friends.

Their biggest issues were blame, shame, guilt, and

anger. They always blamed themselves. "Why didn't I see this coming? I should've done something … anything!" And then the blame was on someone else, most often another family member. The shame of a family member committing suicide remains with the entire household.

"Why did they do that to me?" It was quite normal for loved ones to take it personally. They felt it was a direct assault against them.

Many felt suicide was a sin and were concerned about how their loved ones would be judged by God, and feelings of despair, depression, and anger followed. Anger at the one who committed suicide, anger at society, anger at everyone. All these feelings are felt by all families whose loved one had committed suicide.

The FOSTER families and I put together a brochure about our group. This is what they wrote:

Please join us in our Support Group for *Families of Suicide to Enable Recovery.*

> Friends and family may not always be able to offer all the support you need. They are involved with their own families and problems of life which are now so different from yours. Even though they want to help, they may be uncomfortable by the death of your loved one who committed suicide.
>
> Grief companions in support groups have been through the valley of the shadow of death. They understand the value of talking and crying together and searching for other alternatives to

reinvesting in life. Linking up with others who have experienced similar losses could provide the emotional assistance in working through your own fears and frustrations. You learn how to be more patient and *more loving* with yourself, your family, your friends. People with similar losses often become second families to each other, reaching out of isolation to a meaningful support system. Just remember, everyone needs help. Don't be afraid to ask, and to accept help when given.

Come to Mt. Lebanon United Methodist Church the 1st and 3rd Monday each month 7:30–9:00 p.m.

As the group grew, many people asked me a compelling question: "Why don't you start a group for people who *are* suicidal? You've got the cart before the horse," they would exclaim.

And that was true. They were attending a support group whose loved one *already* committed suicide, and even though the group was important and helpful to them, why not *prevent suicide?*

# Youth Suicide Prevention Program (YSPP)

Many parents were asking me how to talk with their teenagers about death, depression, and suicide. I wasn't sure either. I had three daughters, and I made many mistakes in my ability to talk with them about different issues.

However, I did know that death, depression, and suicidal thoughts could be linked with anger, anxiety, restlessness, panic, and tension, which could cause that age group major emotional problems.

When I first started the suicide prevention support groups, I had to demythologize myself by breaking down old myths I had learned from some external source.

Myths like the following:

*Myth:* People who talk about suicide don't commit suicide. Fact: Of any ten persons who kill themselves, eight have given definite warnings of their suicidal intentions.

-----------------------------------------

*Myth:* People who commit suicide do not have a loving, caring family.
Fact: A great number of people who are suicidal have very caring, loving families.

-----------------------------------------

*Myth:* Improvement after a suicidal crisis means that the risk is over.

Fact: Most suicides occur within about three months of the beginning of "improvement," when the individual has the energy to put morbid thoughts and feelings into effect.

------------------------------------------

Myth: Once a person is suicidal, he or she is suicidal forever. Fact: Individuals who wish to kill themselves are suicidal only for a limited period. With help from counselors, the person's crisis can be worked through.

------------------------------------------

So, what should I do? Start another support group? Some of the FOSTER members thought I should have a group for depression specifically designed for teenagers.

Where do I find them? I couldn't necessarily ask from my church's pulpit for suicidal people to sign up for a support group, so I put an ad in the *Wilmington News Journal* newspaper.

"Teenagers and Adults: If you feel depressed or suicidal and want to talk about your feelings, come to Mt. Lebanon United Methodist Church Thursday at 7 pm."

I decided to call it "suicidal" because I wanted to see if people would admit they were suicidal. And I added "adults" to the ad, just in case teenagers might not admit to feeling suicidal.

When people arrived, I was ready with a small pot of coffee and tea, and some of the church women provided cookies.

Amazingly forty-eight people attended the first meeting.

However, the newly formed support group didn't go well. I made a huge mistake. I invited everyone, meaning all age groups. There were twenty-two adults over fifty years of age, seventeen teenagers, and nine under the age of twelve, and me, the only facilitator.

It was a very long hour, especially because the adults all told the adolescents their problems were easy compared with being an older adult.

One of the conversations went like this:

Teenager: "I have problems with my boyfriend. He just dumped me, and I'm so depressed. I've tried to get back together, but he is going with my best friend. I hate him. I hate myself. I'd rather die. Maybe that will show him."

Adult: "Honey, you haven't seen anything yet. Just wait till you get older. We have real problems ... not your silly problem of just being dumped."

The elders of the group were chastising the younger set when they told them, "You don't know the real problems of the world. Getting old is horrible. I feel suicidal all the time."

It was then I realized I had to split the teenagers from the adults, or everyone would be suicidal.

It was a captivating hour trying to decide what to name each group. The adults wanted to call their group Adult Depression Group (ADG), and the teenagers wanted to name their group Suicide Prevention.

I asked, "Do you think the word *suicide* is better than *depressed?*

Together, they said, "Name it what it is … suicide prevention!"

The following week, I started two groups: Adult Depression Group (ADG) and Youth Suicide Prevention Program (YSPP).

I added the "youth" part to distinguish between the two.

The Adult Depression Group met every Wednesday at 7:00 p.m. in my office at Mt. Lebanon church. There were about eight to ten who regularly attended the support group that lasted until my retirement, when the mental health organization agreed to continue the support group.

The YSPP (teenagers) group met every Tuesday at 7:00 p.m. Over the eight years the group met, there were about nine to twelve teenagers who met with me on a weekly basis.

I was hoping for another clergy or psychologist would help me facilitate these support groups, but most of them didn't want to be sued, and they were sure I would be sued because someone would commit suicide, and "you didn't stop them."

I was never sued, and there were no fees charged to any support group participants. We never charged a penny to any person or family who attended our support groups.

Interestingly, many attendees of our support groups became members of our church because they felt hope and nonjudgment from other parishioners.

That was one advantage of being appointed by the bishop and cabinet to a church ready to close her doors. Due to lack of attendance, there weren't many people who might judge others. I was so pleased that the church members accepted and included everyone. At the end of my twelve-year appointment at Mt. Lebanon, our membership grew to 453 parishioners. The support group participants and their families and friends made up most of our church's membership.

I was quite proud of Mt. Lebanon when she was chosen as the "Model Church in the State of Delaware."

The *Wilmington News Journal* wrote the following,

> Mt. Lebanon is chosen as the Model Church in the State of Delaware. Under the leadership of Rev. Dr. Marlene Walters, Mt. Lebanon has blended the church into the needs of the community. Today the church sponsors many support groups and other programs to meet the needs in the community.
>
> Suicide Prevention programs reach out to those in deepest despair offering hope and practical help.
>
> Families of Suicide to Enable Recovery (FOSTER) supports families of troubled youths and works with an inter-agency council.
>
> The Best Foot Forward program ministers to women in prison offering exercise, rehabilitation and skill developments.
>
> A Clown Ministry visits nursing homes and institutes in the area sharing the joy of faith. A Nursing Home ministry takes seriously the call to care for the sick and shut ins.

Mt. Lebanon was chosen because of their serious engagement in ministries of social justice and has attendance which exceeds the denominational average. Some would say those churches involved in ministries of social justice, compassion and peace will not grow in membership, and those growing in membership will not be involved in social issues.

Mt. Lebanon is a model church doing both saying, "It can be done!"

What a nice honor for our "little church in the dogwoods," as others described Mt. Lebanon United Methodist Church.

I was sure proud of my parishioners becoming involved in all these projects for our community, showing God's grace and unconditional love.

And our suicide prevention support groups grew precipitously.

Since my time was becoming more and more limited, I thought a buddy system might work, like having a buddy swimming with you. I taught swimming before my ordained ministry, and we always swam with a buddy, for safety purposes.

"Wouldn't it be helpful to have a buddy system for those who feel suicidal?" I asked the YSPP group. And they promised one another that if they felt suicidal, they would call and meet each other no matter what time of day or night.

I prayed it would work. And it did. Not one of our group members tried to commit suicide over all the eight years of meetings. Of course, we had different attendees through the years, but each one promised to call his or her buddy. Many continued feeling depressed but found other ways to reach out, besides reaching in. That doesn't mean it was all rosy. It wasn't. Often, I found myself meeting them in different places, trying to listen to their problems and, in some cases, getting advice from my psychologist friends.

The teenagers really did call one another, meet, and share their problems in between the support group meetings. What's more, the teenagers were bringing their friends to the YSPP group, friends who weren't necessarily suicidal, but they were caring and wanting to learn how to help.

With my new knowledge concerning suicide, I was invited to speak to community groups, and high school classes asked me to speak to their constituents. Sometimes these speaking engagements became a biweekly occurrence.

Several of the young members of our YSPP group began to join me in my presentations. I was always so proud of their courage and openness to discuss their fears, depression, and suicidal thoughts. It's through sharing and caring that healing begins. Together, we went to a variety of school groups, social groups, organizational groups, corporate groups, and television presentations telling the truisms of suicide and how to prevent, especially teenagers, from committing suicide.

I created a brochure on the warning signs of suicidal people, and the young teens helped me prepare it.

We called the brochure, "Is Life a Puzzle?" (It sure is.)

This is what the *YSPP* and I put together as a handout.

Suicide is now the number two killer of young people between ages fifteen and twenty-two. Reported suicides are, however, just the tip of the iceberg. Many deaths that are self-inflicted are reported as accidents or homicides by officials.

The tragedy of an adolescent suicide reaches far beyond the untimely death of a teenager. Parents, siblings, friends, teachers, even communities are often devastated by this ultimate rejection. Many survivors of a teenage suicide suffer severe guilt, depression, unresolved grief, acute family problems, and they are high risk for suicide themselves, nine times higher than the general population.

What can we do to prevent suicide?
First, recognize the warning signs of suicidal people:

... More Withdrawn, uncommunicative and isolated from others than usual.
... Deep depression and feelings of worthlessness.
... Expressing suicidal thoughts, even jokingly.
... A change in manner, some air of giving up that you can't quite pin down, but makes you think, "something is wrong."

… Written material that seems disorganized or has heavy themes or overt references to death.

… A quiet settling of affairs, such as the giving away of prized possessions.

… An increase in cuts, bruises and accidents.

… Persistent boredom and/or difficulty concentrating.

… Running away.

… Drug and/or alcohol abuse.

… Noticeable changes in eating or sleeping habits.

GET HELP. Adolescent suicide is preventable. YOU CAN HELP.

1. Listen. Don't dismiss the adolescent's problems as trivial.
2. Trust your suspicions that the person may be self-destructive.
3. Communicate your concerns for the well-being of the person.
4. Talk openly and freely and ask direct questions about the person's intentions. Try to determine whether they have a plan for suicide. The more detailed the plan, the greater the risk for committing suicide.
5. Encourage the person to seek help from a clergy, school counselor or teacher. If the person resists, you may have to get the necessary help for them.

6. Call the police if the situation is immediately life-threatening.
7. Do not leave the person alone, if you believe the risk of suicide is immediate.
8. Do not swear secrecy to the suicidal person. You may lose a friendship but save a life.
9. Do not debate whether suicide is right or wrong. This may make the person feel more guilty and worthless.

There is nothing more difficult to evaluate than a "prevention" program. During the years after we started the suicide prevention support group (YSPP), we did not lose any participant in our group to suicide.

This fact was printed in the July 4, 1988, *Newsweek* magazine, as they featured our suicide prevention support group. They wrote, "hundreds of teenagers have now joined groups for suicide prevention at Mt. Lebanon United Methodist Church. A few of these kids have seriously contemplated suicide but called their buddy in time."

In 1989, I was asked to present a paper to describe the results of surveys I'd given to the YSPP support group and Rockford Center to the International Association for Suicide Prevention XIVth International Congress in Hamburg, Germany.

The title of the presentation was "The Cultural, Social, and Behavioral Effects on the Adolescents Attending the Suicide Prevention Support Groups," by Rev. Dr. Marlene Walters.

"In attempting to evaluate our suicide prevention support group, a group of counselors surveyed the population of these adolescents. The survey was conducted by our Suicide Prevention Council and given to each teenager who attended the Youth Suicide Prevention support group, and Rockford Center, a Psychiatric Hospital for Adolescents support group. I facilitated both suicide prevention support groups over a five-year period. This study was intended to guide counselors, facilitators, families and teachers enabling them to understand some of the reasons why our youth are attempting to take their own lives.

All youth surveyed participated in the suicide prevention support groups four times or more, and both the young people and their guardians signed an informed consent agreement. There were a variety of cultural and social differences in terms of age, family structure, race, environment and training. In all, 997 participants completed the survey.

However, some significant commonalities were unveiled in the study.

The survey to the teenagers asked the question, "does the support group help? If so, how?"

The responses were, "yes," Seventy-eight percent.

"How does the support group help?"

1. People listen. Seventy-five percent.
2. We can express our feelings openly. Seventy percent.
3. It helps to know others have the same problems, Seventy-two percent.
4. We participated in the 'buddy system' where we could call one another when we felt we needed help or want to "just talk." Seventy-six percent.

Other commonalities of the teenagers included:

Sixty-five percent surveyed felt they lacked coping skills and wanted to learn coping mechanisms.

Sixty-two percent wanted someone to listen to their problem.

Fifty-five percent had real or imagined fears of failure.

The most alarming statistic was the answer to the question, "did you have any losses, death, divorce or separations in your family over the past two years?"

Alarmingly, *eighty-two percent* had lost a significant person in their lives in the past two years.

The companion question to this question of "did you suffer any loses?" was:

"How do you cope with your losses?"

A startling *seventy-eight percent* said they coped in this order:

1. Alcohol
2. Drugs
3. Suicide

Those were the top three coping mechanisms the young teenagers used.

These coping tools of alcohol, drugs and suicide are certainly not ones that we, as a society should condone. We need to teach new ways to cope with our adolescents' difficult losses."

As the article in the *Wilmington News Journal* states in its coverage of our suicide prevention support group, entitled: "No Easy Answer to a Child's Pain,"

"There's no single reason children kill themselves. The children might feel abandoned or depressed. They might be angry or feel responsible for a family conflict or divorce. They might be pressured by a hectic schedule, school or peers. They might entertain fantasies about visiting a dead relative. A few might hallucinate or hear voices. Suicide by children shocks society because "we don't think they can be in that much pain that death is something they can wish for." Often the problems seem minor to adults, but to kids, the problems are major. Children may be trying to escape from an intolerable situation at home. They might have suffered abuse, or they may feel pressured by a hurried schedule. Suicide is so hard to predict because a child with a safe home and regular meals can be suffering while a child living in an abandoned building might survive."

My hope and prayer is that we'll learn to deal with these vital issues of death, divorce and separation, so when they happen to our children, we can teach healthy coping methods while the overwhelming grief is still fresh and not yet obliterated by negative defense mechanisms such as alcohol, drugs and suicide.

Therefore, I started yet, another Support Group.

## SUPPORTING K.I.D.D.S. (Kids Involved with Death, Divorce and Separation)

It was at that time I invited a variety of agencies, nurses, psychologists, counselors, schoolteachers, guidance counselors, to see if they might be interested in investigating the importance of a project to help guide families to learn how to cope with their divorces, deaths and separations.

In February of 1989 forty people met at Mt. Lebanon United Methodist Church, including our youngest school teaching daughter, Carrie.

For many months we met and developed programs for all age groups.

We called the group: SUPPORTING K.I.D.D.S (Kids Involved with Death, Divorce, Separation). We refined a training program for facilitators. Four psychologists, six elementary school teachers, four nurses, and three school counselors led the groups.

One night we met for divorced and separated families. We structured the groups in this manner: Children four to six were in a group with a trained facilitator. Ages seven to ten were in another group. Ages ten to twelve; and thirteen to eighteen completed the children's program. The adult group consisted of parents, grandparents and other family members.

On another night, we had the same style groups but for families who were grieving over a death of a family member. All the groups met at Mt. Lebanon United Methodist Church. I facilitated the adult family members who were going through a death.

Now I have no nights open to be with my beloved patient supporter, Thomas J. Walters. Fortunately, our children are adults and are in their professions. And my dear husband brought food from Arby's that we ate in my office at Mt. Lebanon almost every night I had all the support groups, A.D.G.; F.O.S.T.E.R, Y.S.P.P.; SUPPORTING K.I.D.D.S.

One thing is sure. We must watch over our children and not avoid our task of helping them to deal with their feelings around the sensitive difficult issues of death, divorce and separation.

If we do not help them, we have placed the primary burden of coping with family change onto the children, who are not yet equipped with that skill. Then we would be allowing our children to bear the psychological, economic and moral brunt of their losses.

Part of my responsibility of our *SUPPORTING K.I.D.D.S.* program was to interview the new participants. Since my expertise was with the death component, I would facilitate the families whose loved ones died. Originally, we decided to accept children ages four to eighteen, who lost a family member through death, but that changed when one family with three children, ages three, seven and nine were speaking to me about the tremendous loss of their husband and father.

I was paying little attention to the little three-year-old girl.

Just about the time they were leaving, the little girl came up to me and tugged at my jacket. "Hey, you, I hurt too!" she pronounced.

I, insensitively responded, "did you fall and hurt yourself?"

The three-year-old pointed to her heart and said, "I hurt too. My daddy died too."

From that moment on, we decided to take three-year-old into our *SUPPORTING K.I.D.D.S.* program.

*SUPPORTING K.I.D.D.S.* groups grew rapidly with more participants in each eight-week session. We had so many people who wanted to join our groups, we had waiting lists.

Of course, there were no fees charged; nor were any of the facilitators reimbursed. We all felt these *KIDDS* needed help and we could see their appreciation and progress.

For all of us, this was enough reimbursement.

===

I'm sure Dr. J. has heard of our groups because we were featured in many newspapers, on television, and through other communications. But I never heard from him about that possibility.

However, anyone who is caring certainly doesn't want anyone to kill him- or herself and would want kids to learn good coping mechanisms.

Maybe Dr. J. read about our suicide prevention and SUPPORTING KIDDS programs and Mt. Lebanon's and my involvement. Dr. J. might've been interested in our church's participation in our community.

Perhaps Dr. J. knew about our support groups and even sent some family members to join our groups.

At least, that's another possibility of why he gave me his treasured Crucifix.

===========================================

# Chapter 12
## Organ Donation

As I became more involved with death and dying, medical ethical questions continued.

It first started as abortion, then infanticide, then euthanasia, and then I was asked to write an article for the *Delaware Medical Journal,* a prestigious magazine read by mostly physicians.

The article is entitled "A Protestant's View of Organ Donation."

I was asked to participate because of my Doctor of Ministry thesis from EBTS Seminary that I described before.

The beginning of my dissertation asks questions concerning the recognition of life on one hand and the decision to conclusively diagnose death on the other. However, many procedures that aim to preserve life may increase suffering.

When is it justified to withhold or discontinue therapy?

Should we donate our organs after death?

When should death be claimed if organs were to be viable?

Quality of life weighs against quantity, sanctity of life against utilitarianism.

At this stage of biomedical ethics, we must look at the life of sciences in social and religious terms as well as clinical. Any judgment the physician and nurse make on their patient will be made through several crucial human moral problems.

I developed and taught an eleven-week course at Eastern College in St. David's, Pennsylvania; Washington College in Chestertown, Maryland; and the Nursing School of Wilmington.

It was during that time I was asked to write an article on a "Protestant's View of Donating Organs."

========================================

**I was quite honored to be invited to write an article about a Protestant's view of the donation of organs. I didn't know another Protestant clergy interested in medical ethics, so I wrote an opinion, my opinion only.**

**My response was published in the _Delaware Medical Journal_, the official publication of the Medical Society of Delaware, Volume 60.**

**Maybe Dr. J. read the article I wrote. After all, he was a physician and certainly read their monthly journals.**

========================================

## A Protestant's View of Organ Donation
### by Rev. Dr. Marlene Walters

What is one Protestant understanding of organ donation in our society today? If life is a gift from God, can we give parts of this gift to others? There is trust in the commonly expressed belief that life is a gift of God. However, some theologians are not content with the implication of this familiar idea and find some deficiencies. Does the giver of the gift of life require anything of the recipient? Definitely.

Life is not a gift without strings attached. This means that such moral imperatives as justice, love, and compassion are not virtues suddenly invented and added onto life; rather they define what it means to be human.

Life is more accurately thought of as a loan than as a gift from God. For Christian faith, human life is inescapably a moral life, depending on the physiological process of the body, but far transcending it in the dimensions of the soul, spirit and mind.

Then does the Christian belief in the resurrection of the body place any obstacles in the way of a destruction to the body through the donation of organs? Some Christians hesitate to donate their bodies because of their belief in the resurrection. St. Augustine's essay, De Sura Pro Mortius, explains to the satisfaction of most Christians, the answer to this polemic question. At no point in this defense of burial does Augustine make the practice of burial a condition of the resurrection, as though God were somehow prevented from accomplishing His purposes with those who were smashed to pieces or incinerated. Burial, he asserts is "no aid to salvation," but "an office of humanity." Burial is simply a fitting testimony to the resurrection; it does not condemn the body or devalue it to the position of a disposable cartridge.

From this perspective, Christian faith in the resurrection does not present an insurmountable obstacle for the extraction of organs from the donor. Similarly, sharing the loan of our life is a familiar theme for Christians. Just as Jesus laid down His life for us, we are called to demonstrate this similar love for others. Even before Jesus, Hebrew ethics considered the question of the highest commandment. Jesus, faithful to that tradition, made love the supreme commandment, that includes all others within itself. Therefore, love makes no distinction between more precious and less precious, quality or non-quality of life. Every human life is a part of the human community that bestows and protects the life of its members. Jesus said, there is no greater love than that involved in laying down one's life for another (John 25: 12, 13).

Thus, the final loan of our physical body can be given by donating organs to another person as an uncomplicated common denominator of our love and our final outreach to one another. However, as previously stated, our responsibilities for God's loan of our life are the moral and religious imperatives of justice, love and compassion.

How can we apply these imperatives to organ donation? There are several issues in need of continuous evaluation.

## Organ Procurement

How should the organs be allocated? Some have advanced the theory of a free market allowing an international brokerage in cadaver organs. In this market individuals are to be offered financial inducements for the donation of their organs, the price of each organ to be determined in the open market through bidding.

Basically, most Christians would be opposed to instituting a free market such as this on the basis it might lead to injustice favoring certain elite persons in the bidding to obtain scarce organs.

It must be repeatedly stressed that it is the pride of the Judeo-Christian tradition that the weak, defenseless, powerless, unwanted and poor are cherished and should be protected as our neighbor in greatest need.

Therefore, love and caring for all humans, regardless of their condition, are vital guidelines for the procurement of organs. These guidelines were exampled in Jesus, as the empowering disposition to serve another without thought of any good that may accrue to oneself.

Fortunately, the congressional decision to enact the Organ Procurement Act of 1984 bans the sale of organs for the purpose of transplantation. However, the issues of cost, priority, definitions of death and other incentives were not addressed.

## Cost

It is not possible to put a price on life. Even if this could be done, such a practice would corrode the bonds of community that are the cement of social cohesion in every society. Equitable access of patients to organ transplantation should not be impeded by unfair financial barriers.

In the Biblical context of justice and fairness, all transplant procedures that are efficacious, should be made available to all patients through a publicly funded program for patients who are without insurance. This should remove some of the incentives to solicit either by television appeals, prepayment plans, or underground quackery.

## Required Consent and Presumed Consent

One task force estimates that this year 20,000 people will suffer brain death from trauma.

Only 15% of these people will be organ donors. When the rest are buried, they will take with them as many as 100,000 transplant able organs. The same study group proposed a solution: A required request system in which ICU staff were to propose organ donation to families of brain-dead patients. The program was a success, as it increased organ donors.

Others have suggested a weaker required request. This option would help find donors but recognizes the right not to donate and allows for option-out by family members. Presumed consent means that families should be asked, not for consent to the donation of organs, but whether they have any objections. Thus, informed consent is now presumed, making it relatively coercive as compared to the more classical freedom of choice that has characterized our society.

In all consent situations, ethical issues need to be constantly addressed. Are the wishes of donor and family being followed? Are health care professionals making only perfunctory attempts or invoking therapeutic waivers? In order to form an ethical system of checks and balances, and adequate data collection, monitoring the rights of the donor's family is essential to assure trust and support in the community.

Since organ transplants depend on a donor, and the need for organs far exceeds the supply, education is one of the key tools for closing the gap.

Recently, the Delaware Valley Transplant Program, in response to Organ Transplant Week, asked churches and synagogues to distribute brochures on one of their worship days in April or May. At my church on Sunday April 24, 150 brochures were dispensed along with my message on organ donation. Ninety-two parishioners returned their organ donor cards, pledging to become organ donors. Therefore, continued education to all segments of our community can prove to be effective.

## Definition of Death

One of the dilemmas in obtaining donor organs is the controversy over what constitutes death. At the turn of the century, the medical definition of death was by placing a mirror under the nose of the patient to observe signs of respiration. Not too long ago, the traditional view was the absence of a heartbeat. Notice, these definitions were medical and not in the law books.

However, in many states, including Delaware, death is now legally defined as "an irreversible cessation of function of the entire brain, including the brain stem."

The primary reason for legally defining death is to assure that organs for transplantation will be available at the earliest moment and while they remain in a healthy and viable state.

There are two important ethical questions constantly in need of re-evaluation.

First, by redefining death to ensure vital organs are available, are we subtly shifting our attitude favoring the patient as a donor of organs, rather than as a person who may be helped medically or allowed to die peacefully? Legislation could tilt in favor of the recipient rather than the patient-donor.

Secondly, will the definition of death be redefined to include other vegetative persons, who although not brain dead, are in persistent vegetative states? (PVS)

Many medical personnel, and legislators are debating these questions and legislation in several states favors discontinuing treatment for those in persistent vegetative states, therefore expanding the definition of death.

This opens up the question of judgment of quality of life over sanctity, usefulness over worthlessness.

These new definitions of death evoke at least six questions for continuing evaluation by our entire society.

1. The moral domino or slippery slope theory: will more laws open the door to active euthanasia?
2. The Protestant theologian, Joseph Fletcher said, "the act of omission is the same as the act of commission." Therefore, will it be more humane to actively euthanize the hopelessly irreversible ill to alleviate their suffering?
3. When is an illness in fact irreversible or hopeless?
4. Does hopelessness connote meaninglessness, thus inhibiting the use of prudentially justifiable therapy for the seriously ill?
5. Will those responsible for not feeding people in persistent vegetative states always act in the best interest of the patient, thus depriving the patient of some safeguard against human caprice?
6. Cyclosporin and other anti-rejection drugs are rendering more successful transplants. This may mean removing organs at once eventually might not compromise the quality of these organs. Harvesting organs will be technologically possible in the near future. Should this happen, will we eliminate from our law books the definition of brain death that was written to "assure organs would be available at the earliest moment?"

If we continue legally defining brain death as a flat EEG, will we then be able to legally define when life begins as a normal EEG? If so, that would mean a baby eight weeks in the pregnancy is alive, and a person with all the rights of a human being.

These questions need ongoing deliberation and entrapment.

## Conclusion

This is not an exhaustive Protestant prospective, because there are too many Protestant denominations all with varying governing policies.

However, the apex of the Christian faith is the perception that the suffering that accompanies all parts of society can be overcome by the divine sharing of it. The main thrust of the cross in Christian faith appears to agree with the purpose of such applied scientific techniques as organ transplantation. Both the cross and organ donations argue for the preservation of life. However, as history has shown, even the best purposes can be corrupted.

Therefore, the moral and religious imperatives of justice, love and compassion need to be continually interfaced with the ongoing debates concerning all medical ethics.

What were the religious imperatives of justice, love and compassion in the Christian communities?

For the Christian community, it is the injunction of scripture to love your neighbor as yourself ... the sick is a neighbor ... the dying is the neighbor.

The ultimate covenant incorporating justice, love and compassion should be an ongoing dialogue with laity and professionals so that we work together in building trust and cooperation with one another because greater love has no one than this: to give our life for our friend (John 15:13).

==========================================

**Dr. J. didn't comment on my organ donation article, but it's a great possibility he read it. I'm certain, at one time or another, he had to question organ transplanting in his large pediatric practice.**

==========================================

# Chapter 13

## The Act of Omission
## Inactive Euthanasia—Hospice

Let me ask you something.

How would you feel taking care of this patient? The patient is a male who appears his reported age. He neither speaks nor comprehends the spoken word. Sometimes he babbles incoherently for hours on end.

He is disoriented about his person, place, and time. He does, however, seem to recognize his own name. I have worked with him for six months, but he has not recognized me in this time period.

He shows complete disregard for his physical appearance and makes no effort whatsoever to assist in his own care. He must be fed, bathed, and clothed by others. Because he is edentulous, his food must be pureed, and because he is incontinent of both urine and stool, he must be changed and bathed often.

His shirt is generally soiled from almost incessant drooling. He does not walk. His sleep pattern is erratic. Often, he awakens up in the middle of the night, and his screaming awakens others.

Most of the time, though, he is friendly and happy. However, several times a day, he gets quite agitated without apparent cause, and then he screams loudly until someone comes to comfort him.

How would you feel taking care of this person? Or is this a person? Would you feel frustrated, angry, disappointed, and upset and want to quit trying. Perhaps you'd like to throw in the towel saying, "What's the use?"

You would feel all these negative emotions. I know I did.

But I got over it because I was taking care of my six-month-old grandson.

Why is it so much more difficult to care for a ninety-year-old than a six-month-old with identical symptoms?

We need to change our perspectives. The aged patient is just as lovable as the child. Those who are ending their lives in the helplessness of old age deserve the same care and attention as those who are beginning their lives in the helplessness of infancy.

Yes, we elders need to be loved just as we needed love in our infancy.

In fact, because we lose spouses and friends as we age, our needs are magnified, and our losses are daily.

My beloved mom was 105.5 years old when she died. She experienced, as I'm now experiencing, daily losses— loss of eyesight, hearing, sense of smell, friends who are dying, as well as loneliness, sadness, and worthlessness, as we wait for the grim reaper, as some of our friends call "it."

It's not easy to grow gracefully as we age.

There's also the societal attitude that should you get sick, it would be better if you didn't linger. After all, who wants to suffer, especially when you're old and death is around the corner? Why prolong it when sickness comes?

No one wants to be a burden.

Should we allow people to choose when they have a right to die? It's difficult to oppose a person's right to self-determination concerning decisions about treatment.

However, we must take into account that a significant fraction of patients pronounced terminally ill by their attending physicians survive for a much longer period of time than predicated. Just look at the statistics from people who have been in a hospice. Two doctors have to proclaim the patient has six months to live, but many live longer than six months, and I wonder, what if we had given the patient who lived longer some extraordinary medical care? Is there a possibility that person might've lived much longer than the projected six months?

When I was at the medical center, I became involved with an oncology team of social workers, dietitians, nurses, physical and occupational therapists, and doctors. We met weekly to evaluate all cancer patients in the thirty-seven-bed oncology unit. We were the forerunner of a group called "hospice." The big difference was we made no *final projections* that a patient had six months or less to live. We treated each patient as though they had forever to live.

Hospice is distinctive in the definition as I've taken from their website that says the following:

> Hospice care is a type of care and philosophy of care that focuses on the palliation of a chronically ill patient's pain and symptoms and attending to their emotional and spiritual needs. In the United States the term is largely defined by the practices of the Medicare system and other health insurance providers, which make hospice care available, either in an inpatient facility or at the patient's home,

to patients with a terminal prognosis who are medically certified to have less than six months to live.

The act of omission means excluding or leaving out or doing nothing. So, if you become a patient of hospice, except for pain control, nothing medically will be done. No medical tests and no extraordinary procedures will be performed.

While I appreciate and approve of hospices, as they take care of the patient, even allowing pets in the rooms, beds for family to rest beside their loved ones, pain control, and palliative care, there are questions we need to ask before we choose hospice care.

To the family members and patients, please get two doctors' opinions. When you're meeting with them, ask your doctors these questions:

- At what point in an illness does the emphasis switch from treatment to pain control?
- How do you determine who has six months or less to live? Does the physician make that decision alone? Or should there be other doctors, nurses, and health-care people to make the final decision?
- If no diagnostic work is to be done when a patient is in a hospice, how does one know whether the palliative care is simply masking the symptoms of a separate and easily treatable condition?
- Might a backwoods physician in another community deem a patient ready for hospice where a more

sophisticated physician would find the patient's condition treatable? Remember, procedures regarded as extraordinary five years ago are viewed as ordinary today.

- Will you, as a doctor, visit me and get an MRI, X-ray, or other medical treatments should I need them? In fact, will you come to the hospice and treat me at all?

While I'm concerned with the no treatment stance of hospice, none can fault the humanistic and supportive goal. To the dying patient, loneliness and isolation are as big a problem as pain.

Why not provide this kind of hospice care to all patients? Those who are taking medical treatment, as well as those who are not taking medical treatment. Let's not limit care only to those with "terminal disease." Since it's been decided, when you enter a hospice program, you don't need any treatment, except for palliative care, why live those extra days or months in pain, distress, physically mentally and emotionally wasting away to nothingness? Why not give them a pill to put them out of their misery?

One of the concerns I have is the probability of hastening the death of one who is labeled "terminal." After all, under hospice care, the decision has already been made that you only have six months or less to live. If the goal is to alleviate suffering, many ask this question: "Wouldn't it be more merciful to hasten the process, rather than let the patient suffer and slowly die over a six-month period of time?"

Hastening the dying process would be active euthanasia,

or the act of commission, when someone gives the patient medicine to die.

Hence, the act of omission, only giving palliative care, could easily become the act of commission, which is called physician-assisted or doctor-assisted suicide.

However, first you sign your Living Will.

========================================

**I don't know how Dr. J. felt about hospice care, but when it comes to the living will, I'm sure he was aware of all aspects of the living will because his wife, "Iris", cosponsored the living will bills in the state of Delaware.**

========================================

# Chapter 14
## Living Wills

Many proponents for "the right to self-determination concerning their decisions about medical treatment" advise you to write a living will. This is a legal document. All you need to do is fill it out and have it witnessed.

Here is a living will that you could sign in advance of any health problems.

### Living Will Declaration

This is an important legal document. A living will direct the medical treatment you are to receive in the event you are in a terminal condition and are unable to participate in your own medical decisions. This living will may state what kind of treatment you want or do not want to receive.

Prepare this living will carefully. If you use this form, read it completely. You may want to seek professional help to make sure the form does what you intend and is completed without mistakes.

This living will remains valid and in effect until and unless you revoke it.

Review this living will periodically to make sure it continues to reflect your wishes. You may amend or revoke this living will at any time by notifying your physician and other health-care providers. You should give copies of this living will to your family, your physician, and your health-care facility. This form is entirely optional. If you choose to use this form, please note that the form provides signature lines for you, the two witnesses whom you have selected, and a notary public.

"To my family, health care provider and all those concerned with my care: I,_____, direct you to follow my wishes for care, if I am in a terminal condition, my death is imminent, and I am unable to communicate my decisions about my medical care.

With respect to any life-sustaining treatment, I direct the following: _____If my death is imminent or I am permanently unconscious, I choose not to prolong my life. If life sustaining treatment has been started, stop it, but keep me comfortable and control my pain.

Date and your signature
Witness.

-----------------------------------

When I taught medical ethics to the interns at Christiana Care Health Services in Wilmington, Delaware, for ten years, I would invite each doctor to write his or her own living will. Even though the preceding living will is the one accepted by the legal system, still the internists did not know entirely how to interpret the document. How would they treat this patient if other medical issues ensued?

"What does the patient really want me to do?" the doctors inquired.

So, I asked them to write a living will that they would be able to enact, if they received this from a patient or family member under their care.

Not one doctor in all those ten years could write a medically sound living will that would cover every medical problem they would encounter.

But some tried.

I've chosen one living will, written by Marya Mannes, author of *Last Rights: A Case for the Good Death*, that attempts to cover every medical situation a person might encounter.

Read it and the response immediately following, and determine how you might write your living will, covering all aspects of how you want to die.

## The Living Will

To: My Doctor, My Lawyer, My Closest Relative, My dear Friends.

I ask each of you, in concert or individually to assure that certain measures be taken to end my life should I fall victim to the following circumstances:

Singly or together, they would deprive me of all that I cherish most in living, preferring death to their loss.

This document to be resigned by me every two years to and until the event that loss of consciousness through accident or illness precludes my signature. In this case, the wishes expressed are to be carried out by the person herein addressed.

1. Any disease or accident that would leave me unable to take care of my own bodily functions or deprive me of independent mobility.
2. Progressive deterioration of mind as evidenced by total loss of memory, only partial consciousness, chronically irrational behavior, delirium or any other evidence of advanced senility.
3. Any condition requiring the use, beyond two weeks of mechanical equipment for breathing, heart action, feeding, dialysis or brain function without a prognosis of full recovery of my vital organs.
4. Any progressive deterioration of muscle, bone, or tissue requiring an increasing dependence on intravenous substances and without realistic hope for recovery consistent with my definition of such.

5. I do not wish to survive a stroke that impairs my ability to speak or move, nor any accident or disease resulting in vision too impaired to see or read, or in total deafness.

A world without beauty heard or seen, is not a world for me.

A life without freedom and movement, is not a life for me.

If age and illness deny me these, I choose death. And if a difference of opinion among you, results in ignoring or only partially acceding to these requested, then I beg that one of you provide me with the means to take my own life while I'm in a conscious state.

Signed _____

Date _____

Witness _____

The following response to Marya Mannes Living Will, was written by a nurse at the Wilmington Delaware General Hospital:

To: all those caretakers who will take care of anyone who signs this Living Will.

In response to the Living Will, Marya Mannes is a real bundle of joy.

She would "do in" even the well cared for. She wants life to march by her door in brisk formation, stepping high and singing loud … or off with your head!

You bet death is a dirty word.

And the anti-abortionists are right. Abortion really does lead to mercy killing and the promoters are using the same language and the same tactics. And the same media is flooding us with the same hard soft sell.

All in the name of "mercy, personal rights and freedom."

As a care provider, I have a few thousand questions to address the signers of the "LIVING WILL," because I may be the one expected to administer it.

If I misinterpret what you sign, or just let my fatigue show near the end of a wild eight-hour shift, I may just shove you into the great beyond before you are ready.

Do you present this document to me when you check in? Do you give it to the gal in admitting so you can be put in a special section?

Should we call this section, Hospice or the End room?

Do I accept it from trusted relatives or from friends?

How do I know who this is?

Will the ones you don't trust, look different?

Do I only follow your doctor's orders?

Suppose she/he takes off on a world tour? Can the resident or intern write in final orders?

By bodily functions, I assume you mean bladder and bowel control. As so few patients following surgery are left with this dignity, does the need for a catheter, or an enema put you in the "worthless" category? How many soiled beds should I allow you before I put you out of your misery ... and mine?

All of us exhibit signs of senility at least once a day, including people who write and publish Living Wills.

Do we put you through a memory and sanity test each hour? What's the passing score? How about two weeks and one hour or two weeks and one day, as the limit of dependence on some lifesaving gimmick? Who does the countdown? What constitutes "full recovery" of vital organs?

Emphysema is an irreversible condition of the lungs, no way can I make this vital organ whole again.

How do I resolve this?

Do I ask you if you've had enough intravenous feedings?

Do we, in committee, decide? Or will there be a standing House order?

And, if I chicken out, can I leave scalpel or syringe or pills at your bedside? What if you botch the job?

Do we all get another chance?

Do I tell you when I bring in the final dose?

Do I insist you take it, even if you change your mind? How do I keep the confidence of my other patients who get nervous with all this insanity swirling around them?

Only a society on the skids, decadent, and economically insecure, gets so preoccupied with "death with dignity."

Abortion hasn't spread enough death in the land, now we're being told we must legalize suicide and mercy killing. Let's outlaw Living Wills and death with dignity and bring back, SANCTITY OF LIFE!

----------------------------------------

I think this response to the agnostic contentious living will written by Mary Mannes, says it all, succinctly and accurately.

As of today, in 2021, federal regulations require every hospital and health program that receives any Medicare or Medicaid funds to inform you, upon admission, of your rights regarding an advance directive. As a result, many facilities are giving patients a living will or durable power of attorney to sign at the time of admission. This is usually a difficult time to sign anything when you're under stress, and there's so much paperwork.

Hence, the admonition is to sign your Living Will while you're healthy and of sound mind.

========================================

**I'm certain that Dr. J. had to be familiar with Living Wills, because his wife, Iris, as a Delaware House of Representatives member from 1979 to 1998, introduced several Living Will bills.**

========================================

# Chapter 15
## "Iris"

Dr. J.'s wife—I'll change her real name to a pseudonym "Iris"—was a former member of the Delaware General Assembly in the Delaware House of Representatives.

I met Iris when I debated her living will expansion Senate Bill 19, which would "give people broader authority to decide in advance how far doctors and nurses can go to extend their lives in the event of irreversible coma or terminal illness."

Iris's bill would allow people to *prohibit/stop* taking intravenous food or water. It would also allow a person to elect a surrogate to make life-or-death decisions if they are unable.

It was a highly controversial expansion of Delaware's Living Wills law, and I opposed it.

Here is my critique of Iris's Senate Bill 19 that I presented:

> To Members of the Health and Social Service Committee,
>
> "One of the legal dilemmas of our electronic age is too much unnecessary legislation enacted too soon and in response to many nonproblems. This is especially true in the legal-medical area, where physicians are slowly being hemmed in by such legislation and find themselves unable to practice their art and to exercise their best judgment in doing so.

The Living Will is a typical example of that phenomenon. Enacting the legislation of Senate Bill No. 19 gives nothing to people which they do not already possess. If anything, it adds officious burdens to the death bed, encumbers medical decisions with unnecessary additional consultations, and creates rather than clarifies legal problems.

As a chaplain at the medical center for eight years, I can verify that patients always had the right to refuse treatment. We never chained our patients to the beds and made them take their medicine or forced treatment on them. It was mandatory to give all patients an Informed Consent for their signature before any procedures or therapies were begun. And, if the patient was comatose or unable to sign, their family members would sign the consent.

If the patient or family did not wish to continue treatment, treatment was stopped, and love, care, and pain control became the final objectives.

So why is this Living Will bill necessary?

Some have argued that Living Will legislation is the opening wedge toward the ultimate legislation of euthanasia. Since this legislation adds nothing to the legal rights people already possess under the law, nor gives physicians additional protection not already possessed, there may be some truth to this charge.

The bill also gives the impression that decisions concerning the means used to prolong life in danger of death can be made in a routine, abstract, or impersonal manner.

These decisions are not automatic: they cannot be made according to a general rule that applies to all individuals regardless of age or illness. Every situation is different so there will need to be decisions which consider each person's circumstances.

A person could change his or her mind between the time the Living Will was signed and the time of the danger of death.

If an elderly or infirm patient had signed a Living Will, would his or her family and physicians later consult him or her concerning the decision to prolong life?

Voluntary consent is a difficult problem, and Senate Bill No. 19 doesn't make that problem any easier. In fact, it compounds it.

For example: Section 2501: uses language that conditions the validity of the directive to a voluntary consent given, "when the patient was of sound mind." How in the world can a physician know if, when signing the Living Will, whether the patient was of sound mind more, than if they wished to revoke the will when it became apparent death might be imminent?

A far more important problem created by the act and one which might surprise its sponsors, is that the act will inhibit rather than increase the physician's ability to solve with dignity and grace the problem of the dying patient.

Anytime a statute is passed regulating conduct and creating rewards and punishments for noncompliance, such an act has the effect of chilling or inhibiting similar conduct otherwise legal. Consequently, even though Section 2507 is in the act (when the patient was of sound mind), still the effect of the act will be to chill and inhibit otherwise lawful conduct of a physician in withdrawing life-sustaining means, unless such a Living Will has been made by the patient. The physician will assume that he or she cannot withdraw life-sustaining means unless such a Living Will has been made by the patient in compliance with the act.

In the State of California, since their Living Wills were enacted in 1976, which Senate Bill 19 simulates, several physicians testified at their Senate committee on Aging, that two standards of treatment are now being used.

First, under-resuscitation of the patient who *has* a Living Will.

Second, over-resuscitation of the patient who does *not* have a Living Will.

Therefore, the Living Will bill, from the point of view of the physician who has been trained to preserve life, he or she now is in the ominous position of peer-review for actually *providing* treatment to a patient.

How can the physician adhere to the Hippocratic oath under these circumstances? Decisions as to what constitutes ordinary and extraordinary means of prolonging life must depend upon the person and the circumstances of each case.

Specific treatments or drugs cannot be designated as ordinary or extraordinary unless the details and the conditions of the case are known. Penicillin is not an ordinary means to prolong life for people who are allergic to it. Usually, oxygen is considered an ordinary means, but a patient on a respirator may not consider it ordinary.

If the Living Will becomes legal and mandatory, the delicate, individualized care necessary when making decisions concerning the prolongation of life, even when patients are not conscious, would be endangered if not eliminated.

Objections to the Living Will also have been expressed by leading physicians. The Living Will implies that all physicians will try all means to keep dying patients alive as long as possible.

Several physicians have testified that this is not proper to their ethos. They are not interested in prolonging terminal cases through extraordinary means. But the simple fact of the matter is that it is often difficult to judge when a patient's illness is truly *terminal*.

As one expert, Dr. Lawrence Foye, director of Education Service Veterans Administration of New York, explained at the hearings before a special committee on aging, "such approaches as legalized euthanasia and the Living Will are based upon the misconception that the point of hopelessness can be known with accuracy and that the physician may uselessly prolong suffering beyond that point. Unless people understand the false reasoning behind these concepts the physician' hands may be tied in just those cases where his skill and modern technology can make the greatest contribution to the saving of lives and the control of disease."

Another shortcoming of the Living Will, more subtle but nonetheless serious, is the atmosphere it creates. A mercenary, cold, and pagan atmosphere surrounds the Living Will itself and the literature supporting its legislation. One of the main arguments in favor of legalizing passive euthanasia or letting someone die by prior agreement, is the emphases on the cost of keeping people alive. This argument conceives that the infirmed are a financial burden upon society; it seldom mentions the contribution they may be making or have made.

Ethically our understanding of this problem must be based upon our understanding of respect for the person. Each person is a unique entity not only in the eyes of God but also in the eyes of the United States Constitution and the criminal law of all our states.

A *dying* person is no *less* a person in the eyes of the law.

Ethically he or she not only continues to be a person of infinite moral worth and humanity, but also, she or he now has a greater claim on us and on our humanity because he or she is ill and helpless.

Even more so, his or her claim upon the practitioner of the healing art is raised to a higher level because of the illness. Each one of us deserves, from each other, the respect we all feel is due to ourselves and never as a means toward an end.

In addition, as each of us exists in this society, we depend upon the covenant that each one of us has with each other: that certain rules of the games ... certain unspoken promises we have made to one another ... will be followed by all of us. One of those rules or promises is that we will not harm one another, even if a person desires to die.

In summary, there are five reasons for opposing the Death with Dignity Bill and Living Wills.

1. The moral domino theory, death with dignity laws open the door to active euthanasia legislation.
2. Difficult defining when any illness is, in fact, irreversible.
3. Ambiguous terms, for example a person who's doing well on kidney dialysis has no hope for complete recovery. Also, technically a diabetic is terminally ill.
4. The fear the "hopeless" connotes "meaningless" thus inhibiting the use of prudentially justifiable therapy for the seriously ill.
5. The presupposition that those responsible for executing death with dignity always act in the best interest of the patient, thus depriving the patient of some safeguard against human caprice.

This Living Will bill is a suicide note, and we the public and even family members will assist each other in that unethical practice.

Blessings, Rev. Dr. Marlene Louise Walters"

------------------------------------------------

Unfortunately, in a 21 to 16 vote, the lawmakers approved this senate bill.

However, as I predicted, once you allow one piece of legislation to open the gates of "death with dignity," Hannah, bar the door ... there will be more!

Not long after, Senate Bill 341 was introduced.

The Advance Health Directive Act Bill 341 provides a method for Delawareans to stipulate their healthcare wishes. S.B. 341 will amend Chapter 25, Title 16, of the Delaware Code, relating to health-care decisions. In broadening Delaware law, it would permit patients to make decisions regarding situations not clearly covered by many statutes, including life-sustaining treatment, artificial nutrition and hydration, and cardiopulmonary resuscitation. Advance Directives allow patients to decide ahead of time what type of care they want. An Advance Directive also allows the patient to name someone else to make health-care decisions.

The year was 1994, and I was asked by the *Wilmington News Journal* to write a commentary about my opposition to this argumentative, disputable suggested piece of legislation.

This bill would allow for voluntary euthanasia, as my article in the *News Journal* June 5, 1994, states.

The headline is "Should Delaware Expand Choices for Terminally Ill Patients? My answer: NO."

Written by The Rev. Dr. Marlene Walters, pastor of Mount Lebanon United Methodist Church, teacher of medical ethics for the

Adolescence Medicine Fellow Program at the Medical Center of Delaware

Does Senate Bill 341 provide for voluntary euthanasia? Yes! And I oppose it for five reasons.

First, S.B. 341 sets forth a legal form whereby a person may appoint an agent, who may, among other things, "direct the provision, withholding or withdrawal of artificial nutrition and hydration and all other forms of health care."

If you sign this form to request the removal of artificial food and water, you will not die a "good death." According to many doctors, taking away liquids would result in renal failure, causing a lingering death that would take days, perhaps longer.

The bill is masked as "patient choice." Legislative approval of certain death by starvation and dehydration signals a willingness of lawmakers to give the go-ahead to lethal injection, which accomplished the same purpose in a more cost-efficient manner.

The "father" of euthanasia and situational ethics, Dr. Joseph Fletcher, said, "the Act of Omission is the same as the Act of Commission. Therefore, won't it be more humane to actively euthanize the hopelessly irreversibly ill to alleviate their suffering?"

Secondly, laws providing for "death with dignity" or "assisted suicide" may lead to legislation permitting euthanasia of congenital idiots, or the mentally ill or persons with Alzheimer's disease.

Will those responsible for not feeding or giving liquids to people in a persistent vegetative state always act in the best interest of the patient? Doctors often need to use mechanical equipment to force feed food and water essential to stabilizing the patient. Recovery time is frequently months. How long will the patient be allowed to be in a vegetative state?

Will the agent appointed by the patient to make decisions about withdrawing nutrition and hydration be able to understand the medical situation? Do we accept euthanasia laws from other states? If Michigan passes an assisted suicide bill, what will Delaware do? And what of a faulty diagnosis? Medical people are fallible. Even if the diagnosis is correct, some measure of relief may be experienced if recovery is given enough time.

In fact, when is an illness irreversible or hopeless? Standards change and new technology and knowledge are acquired, making it impossible to set a criterion defining death.

Thirdly, if S.B. 341 becomes law, will the chronically ill view themselves as unnecessary burdens draining society's limited resources and sign a form authorizing withdrawal of treatment as "the only decent thing to do"? Their motivation would be concern for family and their suffering if their death is protracted.

People may choose death not because they feel their life is too burdensome, but because they view themselves as a burden to others. Especially vulnerable would be the old and institutionalized. Even though they have signed a document, as provided for in S.B. 341, that will not guarantee that their request will be an authentic expression of what they want for themselves later.

What people anticipate they *will* want and what they actually *do* want, when confronted by death, can be the opposite of their initial decision.

Fourthly, S.B. 341 might come to be viewed as the answer to tough medical cases. Rather than focusing on the need for improved treatment for pain and improved health care systems, might we feel that we already have, in S.B. 341, the answer to burdensome medical cases?

If this bill is enacted, don't be astonished to see increasing reliance on it for handling "difficult" cases, along with an increasingly liberal understanding of what constitutes a "difficult" case.

Consider the dramatic change in attitudes toward abortion that resulted from its legalization and the consequent acceptance of abortion as virtually the standard mode of dealing with unwanted pregnancies.

Fifthly, one of the main arguments in favor of legalizing passive euthanasia, letting someone die by previous agreement, is the emphasis on the cost of keeping people alive. This argument conceives the infirm as a financial burden on society.

S.B. 341 delivers the message that "dying can be so bad that you'd better sign a document now rather than face the horrors that await you later." If available pain control methods were legalized, we would not need S.B. 341, Living Wills, or Dr. Jack Kevorkian as our "choices."

The least we must do is debate these issues with community representatives reflecting all segments of society. Let's alleviate suffering through pain medication, love, and compassion instead of "letting go" of the patient and acting as if death is not merely the last enemy but the *only* enemy.

Blessings, Rev. Dr. Marlene Louise Walters

Unfortunately, the lawmakers passed this bill that gives Delawareans broader authority to decide in advance how far doctors and nurses can go or not go to extend their lives in the event of irreversible coma or terminal illness.

Representative Iris, Dr. J.'s wife, who was a primary cosponsor of the bill, said, "This is clearly a very difficult discussion for all of us, especially in an election year."

I'm unsure of why "an election year" was so important, except that her constituents wanted this bill to pass, and "Iris" didn't want to lose her election. What a questionable way to make vital ethical decisions.

Following these bills, another one was presented to the Delaware State Senate 130th General Assembly: S.B. 526, also cosponsored by Iris, the wife of Dr. J.

> An act to amend Chapter 17, title 24, Delaware code relation to determination of death.
>
> Be it enacted by the General Assembly of the State of Delaware.
>
> Section 1. Amend Chapter 17, Title 24, Delaware Code by adding a new Sub-chapter X which new Sub-chapter shall read as follows:
>
> SUB-CHAPTER X. DETERMINATION OF DEATH.
>
> 1795. Definition
>
> An individual who has sustained either (1) irreversible cessation of circulatory and respiratory functions, or (2) irreversible cessation of all functions of the entire brain, shall be considered dead. A determination

of death shall be made in accordance with accepted medical standards.

1796. Immunity

(a) A physician who decides for death in accordance with 1795, is not liable for damages in any civil action or subject to prosecution in any criminal proceeding for his acts or the acts of others based on that determination.

(b) Any person who acts in good faith in reliance on a determination of death is not liable for damages in any civil action or subject to prosecution in any criminal proceeding of this act.

Section 2. If any provision of this Act is held by a court to be invalid, such invalidity shall not affect the remaining provisions of the Act, and to this end, the provisions of this Act are hereby declared to be severable.

## Synopsis

This Subchapter is intended to provide a comprehensive statement for determining death in all situations by clarifying and codifying the law in this regard.

---

Of course, this Senate Bill 341 passed too.

Well, now that we know what the *determination of death* is and how we can extend our living wills, I'm concerned that older people could be pressured to sign the living will before they know what medical problems they might face.

A healthy person may feel strongly that she or he would rather be dead than sustained by life support, but when that day comes, his or her feelings may be different. A living will can be revoked, but that may not be possible if a person is semiconscious, heavily sedated, or unable to speak or is surrounded by uncaring family members.

It is not a great logical leap, given human nature, to suggest that availability may lead to encouragement, which may lead, in turn, to the irresistible expectation that I should not attempt to live, given any form of diagnosis that is thought to be terminal.

And, what about a flat-lined or flat electroencephalogram (EEG) that measures your brain activity?

Most people think of a coma as a state of limbo between life and death. The word *coma* conjures up an image of a seemingly lifeless patient, hooked up to every mechanical device available. The most recognizable of these devices is the EEG, which measures the brain activity of the patient.

Medical professionals have long accepted that a flat EEG indicates an irreversible coma, one of the most serious types of comas. Furthermore, a flat EEG is often an indication that the brain is no longer alive.

Importantly, new evidence may refute that belief.

The accepted medical definition of a coma states that patients in a coma are in a state of unconsciousness and cannot respond to normal stimuli.

A research team at the University of Montreal found evidence that there are still some traces of cerebral activity in irreversible coma patients. The data gathered from the experiment leads to several conclusions.

Florin Amzica, associate professor of neurology and leader of the research team at the University of Montreal, wrote,

> "First, the research team determined that even when diagnosed with a flat line EEG, the brain is still capable of cerebral activities. A flat line EEG indicates a lack of cortex activity, rather than a lack of brain activity. In addition, the discovery of Nu-complexes points to the ability of the hippocampus to send information to a non-responsive cortex. The researchers propose that the activities from the hippocampus may be a self-protection system. Similar to the way an unused muscle atrophies, the brain may suffer more damage by remaining inactive.

As a result, the hippocampus may send signals to the cortex in order to maintain a minimum activity level, reducing the atrophy that might occur under a long coma. It may be rather useful to keep a comatose brain in this state rather than in the lighter version of the isoelectric line, because the Nu-complex state generates cortical activities that might prevent synapses from degenerating as is probably the case during the flat line."

It's obvious the definition of death is impossible to determine.

Each generation of scientists, doctors, and willing patients that undergo difficult procedures will bring a new definition of when a person is dead.

Once again, it needs to be emphasized, defining death as a flat EEG, or in the early days of no technology, holding a mirror your nose, should *not* be a final decree, as medicine changes as fast as time changes.

Even though a flat EEG is the definition of dying today, tomorrow's new technology might start the brain moving to a normal EEG.

In fact, there is another option to signing the mainstream legalized living will.

The Patients' Rights Council is a human rights group formed to defend the right of all patients to be treated with respect, dignity, and compassion and to work with individuals and organizations to resist attitudes, programs, and policies that threaten the lives of those who are medically vulnerable.

This Patients' Rights group has an advance directive protective medical decisions document you can sign (PMDD). It is a document like the legislative living wills, where you name someone, you trust to make health-care decisions for you. These directives are necessary because federal regulations require every hospital and health program that receives any Medicare or Medicaid funds to inform you, upon admission, of your rights regarding an advance directive. As a result, at the time of admission, you have to sign a living will. Many hospitals are instituting "futile care" guidelines, which may preclude your wishes if you're unable to communicate. An effort is underway across the country to add euthanasia and doctor-assisted suicide to end-of-life options.

The PMDD specifically prohibits *euthanasia and doctor-assisted suicide*. This document will inform the hospitals and medical staff that you want *everything medically possible to be done to save your life* (my emphasis).

That is why my husband and I have signed the PMDD document and have given it to our family, our doctors, and two hospitals where we've been patients: Mayo Clinic Florida and Brunswick Georgia Hospital. We're grateful for the leadership of the Patients' Rights Council with Rita Marker, JD, as their executive director. She also sends

PRC Update monthly newsletters that capture the tone of medical ethical issues in our global world.

====================================

Dr. J. certainly had to know of his wife, Iris's, involvement in these legislative bills she presented, and I objected to.

Dr. J. died in December of 1994, three months after he presented me his treasured crucifix and several months after his wife Iris's legislative actions. He certainly knew both our positions on the living will bills.

Did he favor his wife's Senate Bill No. 19, which allowed people to stop taking intravenous food or water? Or did he favor my objections for opposing the living will bills?

Which one did Dr. J. favor: the moral domino theory- which would open the door to active euthanasia legislation - or the difficulty of defining when any illness is irreversible?

Perhaps he wondered about the ambiguous terms on when a patient has no hope for complete recovery? Or maybe he thought that "hopelessness" might connote "worthlessness"?

Maybe Dr. J. agreed with my questioning SB 19 that those responsible for implementing the death with dignity bill would always act in the best interest of the patient.

Of course, it could be Dr. J. questioned Iris's S.B. 341 that broadened Delaware law allowing patients to decide ahead of time what care they want: an advance directive delegating someone else to make health-care decisions.

Or maybe he realized, as a physician, that the legalization of defining death was not possible, because medicine and science are forever changing.

He must've read my responses in the Wilmington News Journal of June 1994, over five months before he died, December 15, 1994. In that article, I outlined more reasons that I objected to extending the Living Will S.B. 341. I wrote that this bill would provide for voluntary euthanasia that might lead to legislation permitting euthanasia of defective children, infants, and the mentally ill. I questioned the advisability of legislation that might allow those who were chronically ill to view themselves as a burden on society.

It could be Dr. J., being a doctor of pediatrics for over fifty years, still believed in the Hippocratic oath, which calls upon doctors to first do no harm, forbidding abortions and providing drugs for hastening death to their patients.

Did Dr. J. believe in the preciousness and sanctity of life more than the quality of life?

Perhaps he understood my slippery slope viewpoint, that the gradual extension of living wills will widen the groups of patients after it is legally permitted for patients designated as terminally ill. These patients could include people with all kinds of deformities, diseases, disabilities, and mental illnesses and the chronically depressed, and it could permit death without consent.

Did Dr. J. favor my position more than hers? It would be difficult to live together believing in one moral code while your partner believed in another. Yet, many couples who have antagonistic, opposing views are happily married. Not only that but Dr. J. and his wife were presented awards for "their dedicated service to strengthening family life in the community," as Dr. J's obituary stated.

Not many couples receive such a prestigious award.

=========================================

# Chapter 16

## The Act of Commission: Doctor-Assisted Suicide, Medical Assistance in Dying

When a person is close to death, should he or she be allowed to choose death in order to alleviate a lot of misery, suffering, and financial costs?

It's called "death with dignity" or "the good death," taken from the word *euthanasia*. It's an old Greek word, *eu*, meaning good, and *Thanatos*, meaning death. Good-death euthanasia legislators now call it physician-assisted or doctor-assisted suicide or medical aid to the dying.

In the June 10, 1990, *Sunday News Journal*, Perspective insert page, I was quoted about a "Euthanasia" article, entitled, "Facing a Compelling Contemporary Moral Dilemma about Death."

I was asked my opinion about Dr. Jack Kevorkian, who hooked Janet Adkins to an IV and sat back as she pushed the button to release into her vein the combination of drugs that would save her from the degradation of Alzheimer's disease.

It was an act of euthanasia, mercy killing, but technically because Adkins pushed the button herself, it was an assisted suicide. It was a singular event that made headlines across the country.

I responded to the editor of the newspaper, and here is their interpretation of my concerns:

"To some observers, like Rev. Dr. Marlene L.
Walters a Delaware minister with a doctorate

concerning medical ethics, it's a frightening glimpse of the future. The near future, Walters, pastor of Mt. Lebanon United Methodist Church, fears that it is only a matter of time before euthanasia and doctor-assisted suicide are widely available on request to those who are suffering physically or mentally or living lives that lack "quality."

And while Walters has always been something of *a voice crying in Delaware's ethical wilderness,* similar concerns are rising across the country.

Why am I a *"voice in the ethical wilderness,"* as the writer of the News Journal said?

I'm in the *ethical wilderness* because I believe that the taking of a neonatal life, abortion, has opened the medical-ethical door of "court-assisted ethicide," including infanticide, euthanasia, and doctor/physician-assisted suicide.

I haven't met many other people in the wilderness with me, except for the Roman Catholic Church.

The position of the Catholic Church on physician-assisted suicide is fundamentally incompatible with the physician's role as healer and would pose serious societal risks. Instead of participating in assisted suicide, physicians must aggressively respond to the needs of patients at the end of life. Patients should not be abandoned once it is determined that cure is impossible. Patients near the end of life must continue to receive emotional support, comfort care, adequate pain control and sanctity of life respect.

I am grateful there are more voices than my own, in this "ethical wilderness."

Euthanasia, the painless taking of a life to end suffering, has been debated by philosophers, students, and even legislative bodies over the centuries. The case for euthanasia, physician- or doctor-assisted suicide, is based on three central claims:

First, proponents argue that patients whose illnesses cause them unbearable suffering should be permitted to end their distress by having a physician perform euthanasia, or physician-assisted suicide, which is also called medical assistance in dying (MAiD).

The current impetus for physician- or doctor-assisted suicide arises largely because there's so much technology that can keep a patient alive. Because of this, some of the medical professionals give little sustained attention to the possibilities of easing the suffering of dying people, leaving the dying to feel abandoned.

However, the problem of medical abandonment will not be solved by legalizing physician-assisted suicide. The problem may be worsened by such legalization because it could instruct patients and physicians that when death looms, a quick exit is the approved treatment, rather than offering to comfort them with our presence throughout their dying process.

As a hospital chaplain for eight years and a United Methodist clergywoman for forty-five years, I am well acquainted with the blessed relief that death can bring to those who are suffering. But to say that the primary goal is to "hasten dying" rather than to relieve unbearable suffering with pain medication is to blur critical ethical guidelines beyond recognition and to ease the slide toward legalizing physician-assisted suicide.

Second, proponents assert that the well-recognized right of patients to control their medical treatment includes the right to request and receive euthanasia as their basic right. Proponents contend that the right of patients to forgo life-sustaining medical treatment should include a right to euthanasia.

This would extend the notion of the right to die, to embrace the concept that patients have a right to be killed by physicians. But rights are not absolute. They must be balanced against the rights of other people and the values of society.

The claim of a right to be killed by a physician must be balanced against the legal, political, and religious prohibitions against killing that have always existed in society generally and in medicine particularly.

The argument against euthanasia, on grounds of civil rights, involves a consideration of the rights, not just of those who would want euthanasia themselves, but of all citizens.

As public policy, doctor-assisted suicide is unacceptable because of the likelihood or the inevitability of involuntary euthanasia, that is, persons being euthanized without their consent.

Most medical practitioners agree that the relief of pain and suffering is a crucial goal of medicine. The question, however, is whether the care of dying patients cannot be improved without resorting to the drastic measure of euthanasia. Most physical pain can be relieved with the appropriate use of analgesic agents.

Unfortunately, despite widespread agreement that dying patients must be provided with necessary analgesia, physicians continue to *under*use analgesia in the care of dying patients because of concern about depressing respiratory drive.

One of the goals of both physician and advocates of doctor-assisted suicide is to blur the distinction between physician-assisted suicide and the merciful use of drugs that may unintentionally hasten death. This distinction is crucial to the integrity of the medical profession and to the sanctity in which our society holds life. To legalize physician-assisted suicide would be to imperil both ideals.

Such situations demand better management of pain, not doctor-assisted suicide.

Third, proponents are concerned by the frightening prospect that those dying will be shackled to a modern-day Procrustean bed, surrounded by the latest forms of high technology.

Proponents of doctor-assisted suicide often cite horror stories of patients treated against their will. In the past, when modern forms of life-saving technology were new and physicians were just learning how to use them appropriately, such cases occurred, but we have moved beyond that era. Informed consent is now required by every hospital, clinic, and medical facility. Either the patient or a family member, if the patient is unable to bear his or her own witness, has to sign an informed consent on whatever procedure the doctor suggests.

Now, patients may refuse life-sustaining treatment, so doctor/physician-assisted suicide does not need to be an option.

Those who oppose doctor-assisted suicide cite the following four ways in which the legality of physician-assisted suicide could lead to involuntary euthanasia.

The *first* way is "cryphanasia," or a secret euthanasia. The acceptance of voluntary euthanasia may also foster acceptance of involuntary euthanasia and lead to the killing of patients without consent.

The *second* way in which involuntary euthanasia may occur is through "encouraged" euthanasia, whereby chronically ill or dying patients may be pressured to choose euthanasia to spare their families financial or emotional strain.

The *third* way is "surrogate" euthanasia. If voluntary euthanasia was permissible in the United States, it might permit euthanizing incompetent patients based on "substituted judgment" or nebulous tests of "burdens and benefits."

Finally, *fourthly* there is the risk of "discriminatory" euthanasia. Patients belonging to vulnerable groups in American society might be subtly coerced into "requesting" euthanasia.

Historically, the Netherlands was the first European country to decriminalize euthanasia and assisted suicide by a law passed in 2001. The number of individuals who have been euthanized has grown steadily every year, constituting a worrisome cultural shift, which is especially troubling for the most vulnerable in society, according to The News Publications from the Netherlands, November 24, 2019.

Under the Netherlands 2002 Termination of Life on Request and Assisted Suicide Act, doctors may grant patients' requests to die without fear of prosecution, as long as they observe the following guidelines:

- The request must be made voluntarily by an informed patient who is undergoing suffering that is both lasting and unbearable.
- Doctors must also obtain the written affirmation of a second, independent physician that the case meets the requirements and report all such deaths to the authorities.

Dutch physicians typically euthanize patients by injecting a barbiturate to induce sleep followed by a powerful muscle relaxant like curare to stop the heart. Also, the doctor prescribes a drug to prevent vomiting, followed by a lethal dose of barbiturates.

Almost 80 percent of such deaths take place in patient's homes, according to the Royal Dutch Medical Association.

But what if you don't meet these certain guidelines for a doctor to kill you? In the New York Times article April 2012, "Right to Die Push Grows in Netherlands,"

Dr. Petra de Jong leads the euthanasia advocacy group, Right to Die, that cites a case of an eighty-two-year-old man with metastasizing prostate cancer, who is told by his doctor that he does not qualify for euthanasia. The man could contact the Right to Die NL's new "life-ending clinic," and if he appeared to meet the criteria, a doctor and a nurse would go to his home to make an assessment. If all the conditions were met, he would be euthanized, ideally with his family beside him.

Dr. de Jong emphasized that a patient could never be euthanized on the initial visit, because the law requires that a second physician be consulted. The organization is among those pushing to give all people *seventy* years old and over the right to assisted death, even when they are *not suffering from terminal illness.*

Remember when I was at the Wilmington, Delaware, hospital attending Dr. Joseph Fletcher's lecture on "Euthanasia: the Good Death" back in 1970? Dr. Fletcher preached about the importance of dying a good death. "Too much money is spent on the last months of life when the person is dying anyway. Why keep them alive?" Dr. Fletcher boldly claimed.

Somehow, I found my voice and with great gusto said, "Why don't we allow everyone over the age of *seventy-two* to have a choice of living or dying? Perhaps give them a hemlock pill!" I exclaimed.

Little did I know about thirty years later, another country is advocating that very same position, by saying, "all people *seventy* years old and over, should be allowed the right to assisted death, even when they are *not* suffering from a terminal illness."

Not only that but the Dutch position has advanced from euthanasia for the elderly to infants.

Consider the case of a doctor who killed, with her parents' consent, a three-day-old girl with spina bifida, an open wound at the base of her spine. The physician never made any attempt to treat the wound. The treatment was death.

"Euthanasia critics have talked about the "slippery slope" as a possibility; in the Netherlands, it is a fact", according to Wesley J. Smith, author of the book *Culture of Death: The Assault on Medical Ethics in America.*

As the cost of socialized medicine in the Netherlands grew, doctors were lectured about the climbing cost of care. In many hospitals, signs were posted indicating how much old-age treatments cost taxpayers. So professional restrictions against euthanasia have been progressively cast aside.

The Hippocratic oath has either been abandoned or rewritten.

The Dutch Pediatric Society even issued guidelines for killing infants.

> In 1993, the Royal Dutch Society of Pharmacology started sending a book to all new doctors that includes formulas for euthanasia-inducing poisons, according to Richard Miniter, an editorial page writer for

the *Wall Street Journal Europe*. His article, *The Dutch Way of Death*, continues: "Interestingly, the remarkable 33% drop in elderly suicides in the Netherlands over the past two decades coincides with an almost equal rise in euthanasia in the same age group. What Dr. Herbert Hendin, a euthanasia opponent calls, "the Dutch cure for suicide" may simply be evidence of untreated depression.

But, of course, treating depression is costly. If euthanasia began with doctors, it would seem only an awakening of their conscience can stop it now.

An article from <u>Nation & World</u>, Associated Press, December 2004, says,

"Raising the stakes in an excruciating ethical debate, a hospital in the Netherlands—the first nation to permit euthanasia—recently proposed guidelines for mercy killings of terminally ill newborns, and then made a startling revelation: It has already begun carrying out such procedures and reporting them to their government."

The announcement by the Groningen Academic Hospital came amid a growing discussion in Holland on whether to legalize euthanasia on people incapable of deciding for themselves whether they want to end their lives—a prospect viewed with horror by euthanasia opponents and as a natural evolution by advocates. Three years ago, the Dutch parliament made it legal for doctors to inject a sedative and a lethal dose of muscle relaxant at the request of adult patients suffering great pain with no hope of relief.

The Groningen Protocol would create a legal framework for permitting doctors to actively end the life of newborns deemed to be in pain from incurable disease or extreme deformities. Catholic organizations and the Vatican have reacted with outrage to Groningen's announcement, and United States euthanasia opponents contend that the proposal shows "the Dutch have lost their moral compass."

> Cal Thomas, a columnist with the _Los Angeles Times_ Syndicate responded in his article "New Dutch License to Kill a Dangerous Precedent,"

"The Dutch government, which should know better because of its experience with the occupying Nazis, gave physicians their own license to kill. The Dutch Parliament, in a 91–45 vote, set supposedly strict conditions under which doctors may not literally kill their patients. An important line has been crossed for medicine and patients that will not be easily redrawn.

> If there is no Author of life, if there is no reason for curing (i.e., that Man is a unique creation endowed with rights which he receives from a higher source than from the state), then

much of medicine is worthless sentimentality and we could save lots of money, which the healthy could spend, by denying all but the "fit" access to medical care. This was precisely the view taken by German doctors who entered an unholy alliance with Hitler. That experience shows those who will learn from it, that once doctors engage in killing to satisfy a state objective (cost containment, budget balancing, etc.) there will be no limits placed on the use of their skills.

Cal Lewis continues:

"Those who warned of such a progression in the United States when abortion was made legal in 1973 were dismissed as alarmists. That was nearly 40 million dead babies ago. Now we are busy tearing down what barriers remain to infanticide and euthanasia. As with abortion, the hard cases will be used to justify euthanasia, which could then be as accepted by many as is, especially if it is sold as a "benefit" to the younger, healthier and more "useful" overburdened taxpayer.

Shame on the Dutch people for allowing euthanasia to be practiced again in their midst. Are there no history books in The Hague? There is no moral difference between what Hitler did and what the Dutch Parliament did. The empowerment of Dutch physicians with the right to kill is a dangerous precedent which the Dutch people will regret."

But it only took a generation, essayist Malcolm Muggeridge noted, "to transform a war crime into an act of compassion."

Globally, besides the Netherlands, Luxembourg passed euthanasia laws in 2009. Between 2009 and 2018, there were seventy-one medically assisted deaths and more than three thousand people have signed end of life provision forms stating that they want to be euthanized if they are no longer competent to make that choice themselves.

The induced-death practices have become so normalized that on July 11, 2019, the Luxembourg Cabinet adopted a bill that establishes euthanasia or assisted suicide as a natural cause of death.

Canada is a relative newcomer to legalized euthanasia and doctor-assisted suicide, practices that are referred to as Medical Assistance in Dying, or MAiD. The country has so enthusiastically embraced the death practices as normal medical care that since the MAiD law was enacted in June 2016, 13,946 patients reportedly had their lives intentionally ended by doctors or nurse practitioners—in just three and a half years.

With the normalization of medical killing in Canada and the resultant notion that access to MAiD is every qualified patient's right, pressure is now being exerted to force hospices and faith-based hospitals to provide MAiD services even though they conscientiously object.

Not only that but in an Ontario hospital waiting room, they've promoted MAiD by running a public information announcement on a large television screen. The ad shows a doctor's hand resting on the arm of a patient. Below the visual, the following text appears: "Medical Assistance in Dying (MAiD). MAiD is a medical service in Canada, whereby physicians and nurse practitioners help eligible patients fulfill their wish to end their suffering. The text is followed by a toll-free number that patients can call to obtain more information.

Another newcomer to medical killing is the Australian state of Victoria. Victoria's Voluntary Assisted Dying (VAD) law took effect just last year, and it is already apparent that death practices are gaining popularity. They've found a 54 percent increase in people requesting death. In total, 124 died in the first year, with 36 deaths in the first six months and 78 in the second.

------------------------------------------------------------

What about our country, the United States of America?

Surely our doctors, who've chosen their profession to *save* lives, will honor that pledge. Surely our government would *protect* their citizens … all citizens who are disabled, poor, depressed, mentally ill, suicidal, or troubled.

Surely our churches would take *care* of women who

need a group of kind, loving people to help them with an unwanted pregnancy.

Surely people would *reach* out to nursing home patients as they struggle to find someone who cares enough to be with them in their lonely rooms.

Surely God is somewhere in this vast world.

========================================

**Surely Dr. J. saw some of this before his death in 1994.**

========================================

My own medical-ethical journey began in June 1969 with the original abortion bill that allowed women to "abort their fetus if the baby is known to have a handicap."

After graduating from seminary, I became involved in a variety of medical-ethical issues, especially life-ending questions regarding death with dignity, euthanasia, and doctor-assisted suicide.

Amazingly, in a short forty-eight years, our United States of America society has moved to accepting abortion as a standard procedure for unwanted children and to euthanasia for the dying who feel unwanted or lack a quality of life.

Our society has moved very quickly from *birth control to death control.*

There are suicide manuals for terminally ill people teaching you how to successfully kill yourself. The self-help book *Final Exit* features a detailed lethal-drug dosage table and advice to ensure success, such as taking a travel-sickness pill beforehand to avoid vomiting.

In a March 1989 _New England Journal of Medicine_ report, most of a panel of doctors found it morally acceptable for a physician to give patients suicide information and even prescribe an appropriate drug.

Even if the right to assisted suicide were restricted to terminally ill people, it's more than likely that some, especially the poor, elderly, unassertive, clinically depressed, members of disfavored minorities, or some combination of all these would be vulnerable to subtle or not-so-subtle prompting to choose a quick, easy, and inexpensive exit.

If doctor-assisted suicide becomes a legally acceptable alternative to prolonging life, it also will become a cheap and publicly acceptable form of disposing of the more vulnerable of society: the poor, the outcast, and the homeless.

It is far more efficient in society to kill unwanted and undesired people than to care for them with tax dollars in government-funded hospitals, nursing-care facilities, or similar care institutions.

In the United States today, many groups are disempowered, disenfranchised, or otherwise vulnerable, the poor, the elderly, the disabled, members of racial minorities, the mentally impaired, alcoholics, drug addicts, the imprisoned, and patients with the acquired immunodeficiency syndrome.

Many citizens don't have access even to basic health care, and the legalization of doctor-assisted suicide would create another powerful tool with which to discriminate against groups whose "consent" is already susceptible to coercion and whose rights are already in jeopardy.

The Patients' Rights Council, in their July 2019 letter, states: "as of today, eight states and the District of Columbia have changed their laws. They have transformed the crime of assisted suicide into a "medical treatment."

Those states in our country have authorized medical aid (death with dignity / physician-doctor-assisted suicide.)

The following US jurisdictions have death with dignity statutes:

California (End of Life Option act; approved in 2015)
Colorado (End of Life Options Act, 2016)
District of Columbia (DC Death with Dignity Act, 2017)
Hawaii (Our Care, Our Choice Act, 2019)
Maine (Death with Dignity Act, 2019)
New Jersey (Aid in Dying for the Terminally Ill Act, 2019)
Oregon (Death with Dignity Act, 1994)
Vermont (Patient Choice and Control at the End-of-Life Act, 2013)
Washington (Death with Dignity Act, 2008)

Basically, their death with dignity statues, would "allow mentally competent adult state residents who have a terminal illness with a confirmed prognosis of having six months or fewer to live, to voluntarily request and receive a prescription medication to hasten their inevitable, imminent death. By adding a voluntary option to the continuum of end-of-life care, these laws give patients dignity, control, and peace of mind during their final days with the driving force in end-of-life care discussions."

In Washington State, voters are asked to support aid in dying amendments to allow doctors to end lives in a dignified, painless, and humane manner.

In all states, people can only get the medical treatment they want and need if they either have the financial resources to pay for it or if their insurance company will pay for that treatment.

One thing is certain: doctor-prescribed/assisted-suicide is the least expensive "medical treatment." And insurance companies can decide which treatments to cover.

Even in Dr.J.'s and my home State of Delaware they are pushing death on Delawareans. As the Delaware Right to Life _Lifeline_ fall 2021 issue states, "For the fifth time the so-called Medical Assistance in Dying Act, an assisted suicide law Rep Paul Baumbach believes will pass in early 2022. The revised act HB140, is even more sinister than its previous versions, as it makes the "option" of assisted suicide a mandatory requirement to be offered to all terminally ill patients. It also expands who may diagnose a terminal illness to include both doctors and advance practice registered nurses (APRNs)."

In some states where doctor-prescribed suicide is legal, health-care providers are required to inform patients of all options. That includes the option of assisted suicide. According to _Update_, Volume 30, Number 5:

"At the age of 29 Stephanie Packer, a California resident was diagnosed with a terminal form of scleroderma, that can cause the hardening and scaring of tissue in the lungs. Packer is now 33 years old and has outlived her doctor's prognosis of three years more than she's lived.

Recently Packer has been in the news, both nationally and internationally, as a result of a video produced by the Center for Bioethics and Culture Network in which she tells about her struggle with her health insurer to obtain a needed chemotherapy drug prescribed by her doctor. She reports that for five months she's been trying to get on different chemotherapy drugs. She was going back and forth and finally heard from the insurance company that they would cover it but had to check a few things.

But then California's doctor-prescribed suicide law went into effect in June 2016, and her insurance company reversed its decision.

Packer called the insurance company to see why they weren't going to cover the needed drug. She also asked if assisted-suicide drugs would be covered under her plan and was told, "Yes, we do provide assisted-suicide drugs to our patients, and you would have to pay $1.20 for the medication."

Stephanie adds,

> "As soon as this law was passed—and you see it everywhere when these laws are passed—patients fighting for a longer life end up

getting denied treatment, because prescribed suicide medication will always be the cheapest option. Terminally ill patients are "so tired and don't have the strength to deal with the fight, instead they'll take the assisted suicide option because it's easier." (Compassion and Choice Denied, October 17, 2016, on youtube.com)

I was always concerned with people who were depressed and suicidal. Witness my suicide prevention support groups. Now, dismally, that question has been answered by the End-of-Life Option Act.

It's okay to end your life.

According to Wesley J. Smith, JD,'s appraisal in his *Update*, Volume 30, Number 5, article, California: Assisted Suicide for the Institutionalized Mentally Ill.
"Whenever I warn that the same progression will happen here if assisted suicide becomes normalized, supporters of doctor-facilitated death sniff that America is different. But that assurance has already proved empty. California's End of Life Option Act legalizes assisted suicide for the terminally ill who have the capacity to make medical decisions. Please note that having this capacity is *not* the same as being mentally "competent." That implied

conflation is a ruse often deployed in assisted-suicide legalization schemes."

Soon after the California law went into effect, a regulation was quietly promulgated guaranteeing institutionalized mentally ill patients access to assisted suicide if they have been diagnosed with a terminal illness.

Not only that, but the rule permits such people to receive a court-ordered release from institutionalization ... not because their underlying condition has been successfully treated, but for the specific purpose of killing themselves with drugs prescribed by a doctor."

(From 9 California Code of Regulations 4601.)

==========================================

**I can't imagine what Dr. J. would make of doctor-assisted suicide and deciding whether a patient was qualified for being killed, regardless of whether they were terminal or not. I can't understand how any doctor would fall into this abyss. What happened to the doctors in today's world who are enabling doctor-assisted suicide to anyone who wants it? For some patients, they don't have to be "terminal," which we all are, in some degree or another.**

**Would my crucifix-giving friend approve of all this killing?**

**Abortion is killing a live person; infanticide is killing a live person; euthanasia is killing a live person; doctor-assisted suicide is killing a live person.**

**The Ten Commandments from the Holy Bible, Exodus 20:13, say it best: "Thou Shalt Not Kill."**

**Dr. J. died December 1994 after the *Wilmington News***

*Journal* article that called me "an ethical voice in the wilderness."

I wonder if Dr. J. was another "ethical voice in the wilderness?"

Did he agree with me on my observations of the expansion of the living will that his wife legislated?

What did Dr. J. believe? He was getting close to the end of his earthly journey too. When he came to our home shortly before he died, he looked pale and frail, but there he was, at our door, wanting to give me his family crucifix, his personal heirloom given to him by someone special in his family, because on the back of the crucifix are the words, etched in French, "Gage D' amitie " meaning "token of friendship." And inside the Crucifix box was "Cross given to Countess Rehbender to Dr. J. in 1942; given to Marlene Walters by Dr. J. in 1994."

Dr. J. brought me a gift of love, hope, and approval. He gave me something extraordinary that I shall forever treasure.

His crucifix.

=========================================

And now, I'm back to the beginning of my medical ethical journey.

On that infamous drive back to Wilmington from Dover, where the abortion bill was presented, I realized that the issue wasn't just about abortion but the sanctity of life. As a society, we are standing in judgment of all humankind—not just the unborn but the handicapped, the disabled, the misfits, the dying, the reprobates, the imprisoned, the … you fill in the blank.

Who should live?

Who should die?

I entered the ministry because of the abortion issue, but I predicted that the act of abortion would eventually lead to the act of euthanasia. In fact, when I was attending seminary, my husband designed a bumper sticker in black letters against a bright yellow background. I was always proud to drive my old Mustang around with a sign on my back left bumper.

It said, "ABORTION-EUTHANASIA, THEN WHO ... YOU?"

# Chapter 17
## Unconditional Agape Love

On January 22, 1973, I wrote my first piece of poetry and named it

### Where

Where, oh where are the boys and girls today
Who would've been here from yesterday?
The ones whose mothers decided against
Their birth and adolescence.
Oh where, oh where are the
things in the sea?
On the earth and in the air?
The ones pollution did prevent
their tender love and care.
Oh where, oh where are the
people who dissent?
The ones who're jailed for discontent.
The ones who learn by making mistakes.
Room for all we should make.
Oh where, oh where are the
old, sick and maimed?
Their loves, their lives no longer aimed
On life anymore; they're in their place
Tucked away in much haste.
Oh, where, oh what's left on
Mother Earth today?
The perfect person in every way.

The ones who'll obey, learn, and respect
A society that's correct ...
In the minds of a few
Oh where, oh where are the rest today?
They're up there somewhere,
the Good Book doth say,
Where all are welcome in any way.
I'd rather be there ... oh where ...
I'd rather be there.

That poem was written the day that *Roe v. Wade* became the law of the land, January 22, 1973. Today, a woman could legally have an abortion in any state of the union.

It was a sad, ugly day in the life of the unborn, because they'll not be born. Along with some prolife friends from Wilmington, Delaware, on a cold day January 22, 1974, I drove down to Washington DC and joined the March for Life with thousands of people who marched for the life of the unborn child.

Only one other time in my life did I decide to march for a cause. I climbed into a Dr. Martin Luther King Jr. bus from Wilmington, Delaware, to Washington DC on August 28, 1963, to protest the wrongness of the treatment of the African American people in our country. It was at the Lincoln Memorial in Washington that Dr. Martin Luther King Jr. delivered his classic "I Have a Dream" speech. It was another unbelievable and touching event in my life.

I've always been a firm believer in justice and equality

for every living thing: black, white, red, yellow, disabled, infirmed, poor, rich. We are all God's children and loved equally by our Creator.

Although I predicted abortion would lead to euthanasia, little did I know, in my lifetime, that prediction would ring true.

========================================

Time has moved so swiftly that almost forgotten was the loving gift from Dr. J.: his crucifix. On that special day that Dr. J. called to come over to our home on Grubb Road, Tom was facing a terminal medical situation in his life. He had been recuperating from a radical prostatectomy surgically removed by noted urologist Dr. Wein in July 1993. Immediately following the operation, Dr. Wein assembled our family and conveyed the bad news: Tom's cancer was outside the prostate and into the margins. At best, he had three years to live.

Needless to say, our three daughters and I were totally devastated. Dr. Wein added, "We will take his PSA every month, and when it elevates for two months in a row, Tom will need radiation therapy."

I decided to take an early retirement because active prostate cancer usually meant bone cancer, which meant the patient would need a lot of TLC, and I wanted to give him my best. Tom decided to close his successful architectural practice and fight his cancer. After all, who would hire an architect to complete a three- to five-year project if that person had only three years to live?

Of course, we were in a state of disarray when Dr. J. called that morning in October of 1994. Tom had just finished his radiation therapy, and we were getting ready to sell our Walters architecturally designed home on

Grubb Road after living there forty wonderful years and preparing to leave our beloved professions, architecture and ministry. We had not discussed our plans with anyone, so Dr. J. would not have been aware of our new direction.

As Tom and I reflect on the day Dr. J. came to our home and thoughtfully gave me his gift of the crucifix, we didn't realize how sick he must've been and how much energy and thoughtfulness he gave to his journey of passing on his family heirloom to me.

So many years later, after so many life changes, we're finally reflecting on our personal journey and noting the evolution of time and what little time Dr. J. would be alive after he came to our home—just three short months. And just a few months after he died, Tom and I moved to our new home in Chestertown, Maryland, sold Grubb Road, and prepared to retire.

Amazingly, Tom survived his radical prostatectomy and radiation therapy and had now entered a new phase of life: survival. We were elated his PSA monthly readings were labeled "unmeasured," which became our favorite word in the English language.

Tom was fifty-nine years old when he got the three-year death sentence, and he will turn ninety years young this December 2021.

We were so busy with our new life of retirement, we forgot about Dr. J.'s gift until recently, and we began our new journey of searching back to see why Dr. J. gave me his crucifix.

We still aren't sure why I was given this heirloom, but we do know that life is precious, and God is with us throughout our life's journey.

Looking back has provided me the opportunity to ask myself, "Why do I still feel that abortion, infanticide,

**euthanasia, and doctor-assisted suicide are still wrong answers in this ever-changing world of ours?"**

========================================

Tom and I are now in a place that takes care of people in all walks of illness. You name the disease; our Marsh's Edge Retreat will try and take care of you. In fact, Marsh's Edge LLC corporate facility also sponsors the Alzheimer's organization, with all kinds of events.

I'm wondering if doctor-assisted suicide becomes legal in our state, how many people would sign a form that allows doctor-assisted suicide if they are diagnosed with "dementia" or Alzheimer's? How many people would choose to live if they're diagnosed with Alzheimer's, dementia, or a hundred other life-threatening diseases?

What is happening in our country today?

Surprisingly, even the pandemic and the year of COVID-19 didn't persuade people from choosing doctor-assisted suicide.

> What has been happening with doctor-assisted suicide? According to Anita Hannig, associate professor of anthropology, at Brandeis University, in the _Conversation:_
> The corona virus has stripped many of their own deaths, but for some terminally ill people wishing to die, a workaround exists. Medically assisted suicides in America are

increasingly taking place online, from the initial doctor's visit to the ingestion of life-ending medications. Assisted dying laws allow terminally ill, mentally competent patients in ten US jurisdictions to hasten the end of their life. But the move to digitally assisted deaths during the pandemic has enabled other qualified patients to continue to exercise the right to die. In the United States, doctors prescribe a compound of four drugs, digoxin, diazepam, morphine and amitriptyline, to be mixed with water or juice. Within minutes of drinking the cocktail, the patient falls asleep, the sleep progresses to a coma, and eventually the patient's heart stops.

Now, because of the corona virus, volunteers are accompanying patients and families over Zoom and physicians complete their evaluations through telemedicine, based on recommendations released by the American Clinicians Academy on Medical Aid in Dying in March 2020.

Good Grief! You can kill yourself with online help!

Do any groups oppose these new doctor-assisted suicide laws? Thankfully there are some:

American Medical Association
National Spinal Cord Injury Association

World Association of Persons with Disabilities
American Association of People with Disabilities
Euthanasia Prevention Coalition
National Council on Disability
National Council on Independent Living
Patients' Rights Action Fund
Not Dead Yet
Disability Rights Education and Defense Fund
American Nursing Association
American College of Physicians
Roman Catholic Church
Islamic Medical Association of North America
World Medical Association
International Task Force on Euthanasia and Assisted Suicide (Patients' Rights Council)

I thank God for those who oppose doctor-assisted suicide, but there are many who support it, including a Gallop poll that displayed a solid majority of Americans, with 72 percent in favor, support laws allowing people to seek the assistance of a physician in ending their life.

What should we, as a society do?

Should we get rid of those who are in their last years of life and don't want to live?

Should we get rid of the unborn who aren't wanted anyway?

Should we get rid of those born with disabilities?

Should we?

*I wonder.

*I wonder what Dr. J. would think about aborting those born with disabilities.

*I wonder what Dr. J. would think of the Groningen protocol that creates a legal framework for permitting doctors to actively end the life of newborns deemed to be in pain from incurable diseases or extreme deformities.

*I wonder what Dr. J would think about his home state of Delaware HB 140 making doctor assisted suicide a mandatory requirement to be offered to all terminally ill patients.

*I wonder if Dr. J. would believe in doctor assisted suicide. What would he think about eight states in our country and Washington D.C. changing their laws as they've transformed the crime of assisted suicide into an accepted legal medical treatment?

*I wonder how many memory care facilities will close their doors because few people have chosen to live if diagnosed with memory failure, either Alzheimer's or dementia. Most would opt for doctor-assisted suicide.

* I wonder what happens to our mentally ill, our lonely, our depressed people in our nursing homes, and in our State Mental Institutions,

\* I wonder how many Continuing Care Retirement Communities could keep their doors open when doctor assisted suicide becomes a viable option.

\*I wonder what will happen to *research*, when there are few if any people to research because they've chosen to die, rather than live through their disease, enabling researchers to unveil medicinal answers to difficult diseases.

\*I wonder how many not-for-profit organizations will close their doors, because people have chosen to die, rather than live through their disease, no longer needing help from others.

\*I wonder what will happen to the profession of medicine when our doctor tells us he or she believes in doctor-assisted suicide.

\*I wonder how many people will be "chosen" to die, because of their "poor" quality of life.

\*I wonder how many people will die because they were erroneously diagnosed by a world-class urologist predicting they had three years left to live but could live thirty plus more years, like my husband, Tom.

\*I wonder.

Life is precious in all stages.

Each one of us has the gift of passing on our love to everyone we meet. As we say to each other, in our Marsh's

Edge Support Groups, "May the God in me see the God in you."

Of course, we might not feel that way every moment of every day, but with God's love and forgiveness, we try.

How can we pass on God's love when we're ill and dying?

Watch a caring medical person or caring family member or caring friend, and you will witness God's love being passed on.

I have many times.

I watched the lives our daughters Debbie and Becky spiritually change when they stayed with their Nana until she died naturally. Even though she was 105 years young when she died, they were there making sure her lips were not dry, holding her hand, caring for her needs, talking to her, loving her.

That is agape, unconditional love, a love they will pass onto others because they witnessed and embraced God's love of caring for someone who couldn't respond.

We can't explain life before or beyond the points of conception and death.

But the Holy Bible clearly states the love of God exceeds both these boundaries, and that's a process that is open to all of us when we are confronted with a crisis.

We can wallow in the tragedy of it all. We can pull plugs so it will all be over, or we can trust the ultimate grace of God and set out to find the deeper meaning of the experience.

Long ago, a sage observer noted, from Ecclesiastes 3:1, "For everything there is a season, and a time for every matter under heaven."

In other words, nothing happens for nothing.

If we are willing to search, we can find something valuable in every life event. It's not always clear in the instant, but time has a way of revealing a treasure, often in the worst of traumas.

An anonymous Greek philosopher puts it this way: "It is not good for all our wishes to be filled; through sickness we recognize the value of health; through evil, the value of good; through hunger, the value of food; through exertion, the value of rest."

I know that may sound terribly difficult in the shadow of a terminal illness or amid the vacuum of a lost loved one. But remember, our Lord has promised us "we know that all things work together for good to those who love God, to those who are the called, according to his purpose" (Romans 8:28).

As I was frequently in need of a higher Being reminding me that life really is precious, all unborn are human, infanticide is wrong, and euthanasia with doctor-assisted suicide was killing a human being, I was confronted with a situation that I could not answer. Why would a loving God allow this tragedy?

The patient was completely comatose because of a solo car accident. She was not identified by any family members as she lay in the intensive care unit attached to every piece of life-saving equipment that was invented. They called her Jane Doe because the car had been stolen and the police were attempting to locate her next of kin, but she carried no identification.

197

When she was transferred to the ICU, a number of the hospital staff thought she should be allowed to die, and the plugs should be pulled. Some of the staff said, "What's the use? No one is around to love or care for her. What's the point? Why are we tube feeding? Why did the doctors give her a tracheotomy?"

Others weren't sure and wanted me to answer, "Why would God let this happen?"

I didn't know how to answer them, but I suggested we treat Jane as she was, another human being who needed tender love and care from all of us.

As each hospital staff person entered Jane's room to change the equipment or any of the other perfunctory duties they had to perform, each staff member would talk to Jane.

She could not hear, see, or respond.

She was completely comatose.

When I entered her room, I would read inspirational stories from my *Thought Conditioners* or *The Upper Room*.

The nurses and other staff members would tell Jane about their daily activities.

I often heard nurses as they turned Jane and changed her IVs and diapers talking to her. "Oh, Jane, I had the nicest date last night. Let me tell you about our fun together," and each nurse would talk to the comatose Jane.

At staff meetings, they enjoyed telling one another about how Jane was doing today.

It's hard to explain in words how I felt when I heard

the nurses talk about Jane Doe in a hopeful way. I shared that solicitous tenderness that enveloped me, and the staff felt the same way. They too were warmed by their caring responses to someone who couldn't speak, hear, or care.

Something happened to all of us. A miracle took place, one that was indescribable.

We were changed, transformed. For six weeks, we continued this routine, nurses talking to comatose Jane and reporting on her progress "hopefully slowly healing."

Until one morning.

My phone rang.

The nurses were crying. "Jane has died! Oh no! Jane has died!"

At the hospital chapel memorial service for Jane, no family member was there, but all the nurses, unit clerks, phlebotomists, and other hospital staff came.

Each one said words of appreciation to Jane and told of what she had done for him or her.

I sat and listened as each caregiver of Jane Doe came to the pulpit, one by one, and spoke.

"Even though no one knew Jane, we knew her."

"I hope Jane knows we did everything we could to save her."

"Jane listened to me."

"Jane, we'll miss you."

Even though Jane Doe never regained consciousness, we became as one, sharing our love with someone who could not return our acts of kindness.

We were *transformed* as we found love in our heart for someone who couldn't speak, think or give back our love, and we passed that love onto each other.

That's the message that our Lord and Savior brought to us many centuries ago. The mysteries of God's unconditional love as it transcends suffering and agony by touching the soul of every human being who is conceived.

God's agape love.

We experienced it.

We felt it.

We knew God's unconditional love.

As St. Paul writes in 1 Corinthians 13, "Love is patient and kind; love is not jealous or arrogant or rude. Love doesn't insist on its own way, does not rejoice at wrong; but rejoices in the right. Love bears all things, believes all things, hopes all things, endures all things. Love never ends. So, faith, hope, love abide, these three; but the greatest of these is love."

I remained in the chapel after Jane's memorial service, embraced by the sunlight as it reflected the patterns of the stained-glass window—that displayed praying hands, descending doves, the Star of David, the crucifix of Jesus, and, my heart became strangely warmed.

I had received the act of Agape Love from someone who had no quality of life but taught me that life is precious from beginning to the end.

God's gift of unconditional love, a gift that we should pass on to everyone who crosses our path in this journey we call life—the same gift of agape unconditional love that our Lord Jesus gives each of us.

=======================================

**The same gift of agape unconditional love that Dr. J. gave with his Crucifix.**

=======================================

## Life

The holiness of a human life
May revel in love or suffer strife.
Whether in the womb or walking tall
A human life may stand or may fall.
But every life deserves a chance
To sing a song or to dance a dance
To give a hug or receive a kiss
To feel sadness and to cherish bliss
So, when people talk about a choice
And raise a shout with a common voice
May we all make an appeal for life
To spread more love and minimize strife

WHS

Printed in the United States
by Baker & Taylor Publisher Services